Brain & Body Fit After Forty

Moving From Intention To Results

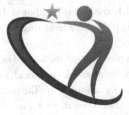

Patrick Streppel

BALBOA.
PRESS

A DIVISION OF HAY HOUSE

Author Credits: Certified Personal Fitness Trainer and Certified Master Coach Practitioner

Balboa Press books may be ordered through booksellers or by contacting:

Balboa Press
A Division of Hay House
1663 Liberty Drive
Bloomington, IN 47403
www.balboapress.com
1 (877) 407-4847

Print information available on the last page.

ISBN: 978-1-5043-6290-0 (sc)
ISBN: 978-1-5043-6291-7 (hc)
ISBN: 978-1-5043-6308-2 (e)

Library of Congress Control Number: 2016911974

Balboa Press rev. date: 08/02/2016

DISCLAIMER AND/OR LEGAL NOTICES

"I dedicate this book to all of you out there reading these words, wishing you an active, independent and healthy life after forty."

Acknowledgements

I sincerely wish thank to thank Gunta Towsley, Mark McAnally and Jim Mavity for their time and patience to read the book, share their comments and give their support.

Most of all I wish to thank my caring, loving, and supportive wife, Denise. Your encouragement when the road got bumpy meant so much to me. Without your continued support I could never have completed this book.

My most heartfelt thanks.

Table of Contents

Preface

Why this book? Why another book about health and fitness, while already so many other books are available about this topic? The short answer is to help you filling the gap between knowing and doing, the gap between intentions and results.

This book helps you to understand the processes in your mind that keep you glued to habits that prevent you from getting the health and fitness results you want. The logical follow-up is that it gives you the tools and strategies to develop and implement habits that support you in achieving your personal health and fitness goals that in turn enable you to maintain an active and independent healthy living.

Of course, expect to read about everything you need to know with regard to healthy nutrition and safe and effective exercising, but I'm not going to leave you with that.

Most books about health and fitness only tell people what to eat or not to eat and what exercises to do, followed by the recommendation to take action and follow through until they have achieved their health and fitness goals, from which moment on it will only be a matter of maintaining.

Reality shows that it hardly ever works this way.

Do you recall that enthusiastic feeling when you thought you had found the book or program you had been looking for? Once purchased you probably couldn't wait to put it into action and see your life change for the better. The reality; after an enthusiastic start and several weeks of hard work you realized that nothing had changed and that nothing was left of all the excitement you felt at the beginning.

From the moment on that book was yours, you felt like sitting in an aircraft with roaring engines, ready for take-off. So why didn't happen what you expected and so intensely hoped for? Simply put and metaphorically spoken, the book or program you had bought gave you the aircraft but didn't come with a runway and a flight plan.

This is where this book steps in. By identifying your personal health and fitness goals, creating a plan to achieve your goals, discovering the options you need to achieve your goals, dealing successfully with the physical and mental roadblocks that prevent you from achieving your goals, you'll have that runway and flight plan that enable you to create the focus, flow and momentum you need to achieve your goals and maintain them for life.

Studies show that 95 to 98 percent of the people who managed to lose weight gained back what they had lost within two years.

This highly frustrating fact causes many people to give up and settle for a life with a body they feel is often in their way. Aside from the physical health problems that come and worsen with every passing month and year as a result of being out of shape, mental problems arise as well that can lead to feelings of depression and living an unsatisfied life.

During my career as a personal fitness trainer I've seen too many people beginning a fitness program with the best intentions, staying motivated for a while and then give up because the results they had hoped for didn't occur, despite all their hard work.

Other people gave up because their hectic life interfered with their workout schedule. After skipping one workout, another followed and so on until they realized that continuing their workout program didn't make sense and that they'd better wait a while for quieter times to arrive.

These are just two reasons why people gave up but a list with reasons could go on forever, ranging from unsupportive family members to setbacks caused by injuries or boredom with the workout routines.

The big question: why is it that only a happy few manage to achieve and maintain health and fitness goals such as losing weight? What distinguishes them from those who keep failing no matter how hard they try?

This question and the will to make a positive difference in the lives of so many whose desperate and rightful goal it is to have a cooperating body that enables them to live a purposeful and rewarding life was the starting point for writing this book.

What I have learned over the years from following, observing and interviewing men and women who had started a fitness program was that those who were more interested in the process than in the end goal had the best papers to succeed.

Of course it was their aim to get the best results in the shortest time possible, but rather than focusing on what the scales were telling them every morning, they were more interested in learning about their body and mind and what they can do to support and stimulate their performance during the fitness program.

Less successful people often tend to focus on the end goal only. It is from these people that I hear comments such as: "Patrick, do me a favor and spare me the details. I really couldn't care less about all that background stuff you're talking about. Can't you just tell me what to eat and what for exercises I should do to get me in shape as quickly as possible and leave it at that?"

The simple question to this answer is no. I learned that when people acquire a basic understanding about the processes that occur in their body and mind, they put themselves in charge of the process with the result that it becomes much easier to make better choices related to nutrition and exercising.

Simply telling people what to do, leaves them with the passive role of follower with the consequence that they can easily become distracted, lose motivation and eventually give up.

Today's society has turned people into followers. Focused on the outside world with all its demands and distractions and a life filled to the rim with responsibilities and obligations geared to the interests of others, many people have lost sight of their own needs and desires.

The result is that once they found some time for themselves, they often leave it to the food, pharmaceutical and entertainment industry what it is they feed and cure their body with and how they spend their free time.

The factor convenience also plays an important role in this context. It is human nature to realize maximum results by spending the least amount of energy. This combined with the high demands of today's society made convenience for many people the leading principle in their life.

Convenience makes it possible to choose for quick fixes at every moment and for virtually every circumstance during a day. Examples of quick fixes are fast food, sweet treats, pain killers and (on-line) entertainment. Whether the motivation is moving away from discomfort and pain or moving toward pleasure and reward, an instant solution with instant gratification is almost always within reach to satisfy the instant needs.

The problem with quick fixes is that they are general, short lived, superficial and come from outside sources. The result is that signals or responses coming from within the body in the form of discomfort or pain with the function to inform us that something is wrong, aren't recognized, let alone understood.

Choosing for convenience and quick fixes is often justified with statements such as "doctors know what is best, and if the food and drugs weren't okay, it wouldn't be allowed to sell them, and it wouldn't be in the shops, right?"

Not even close. The sad truth is that most food and pharmaceutical companies only look after their own interests, and government organizations and health care professionals are barely able to withstand the lobby of the food and drug industry.

The fact that statistics year after year show how overall health is declining while health care expenses are going through the roof illustrates how powerless government organizations, doctors and health care institutions are when it comes to guaranteeing food safety and curing life style related diseases and illnesses.

Another example of how people have turned themselves into followers, succumbing to convenience and quick fixes whenever possible, are the unhealthy diets and unsafe exercise regimes they purchase in order to deal with the unwanted effects of being out of shape such as weight gain and feeling weak.

When it comes to achieving health and fitness goals there is no such thing as a quick fix or a one-solution-fits-all approach. Everybody is unique and improving overall health and fitness begins with understanding and respecting the specific needs of one's body. Any other approach equals wasting time, money and energy and the risk of harming the body.

Taking responsibility for one's health and well-being begins with turning away from quick fixes provided by diets and programs that have no clue about the individual body and mind. The next step is accepting and taking up the role of being the true expert of one's own body and mind.

This book will help you becoming the true expert of your own body and mind. It is not difficult at all and will feel like taking off a blind fold. Step by step you will begin to connect the dots and see yourself taking the steps that already cover half the road toward successfully filling the gap between knowing and doing, the gap between intention and results.

The other half of the road to success is covered by actually implementing the gained knowledge. This is a totally different kettle of fish and one that has proven to be crucial for success.

Unfortunately, here is where it often goes wrong. Reality learns that bringing up the patience to learn how body and mind work already is a big step for most people. Asking them on top of this to put in even more effort to educate and train their mind to establish supportive habits that help to stay motivated and on track toward their goals is often a step to many.

When it comes to making changes, the mind often acts more as an opponent than as a friend. To understand why and what to do to solve this problem, it is essential to learn how the brain and mind function. Without this important first step nothing much can be expected from efforts such as losing weight, regaining strength or any other goal in life for that matter.

To clarify the difference between brain and mind; the brain represents the hardware or physical content of the skull and the mind the mental or software content.

At the time of writing this book, searching for health and fitness quotes on Google produced about 45,200,000 results. Most of them are true and very inspiring. It illustrates that we all know what to do. Fact however remains that 95 to 98 percent of the people are unable to flip the switch in their mind to actually take action and succeed.

For years people have been trying to convince themselves that all it takes for them to succeed this time is by taking once more a firm stand and then just do it.

Problem is that the strategy of just do it relies on a short burst of willpower, whereas the endeavor of achieving and maintaining a healthy lifestyle lasts a life time. Sadly, since not many know of another strategy, most people keep following the same old stale advice repeated over and over in most books, magazines, the internet and some of my colleagues.

Using just willpower is like holding your breath under water. Some may be better at it than others but it is not an effective strategy for making long term lifestyle changes.

What I strive for with this book is to stop people punishing themselves and beating themselves up for not being able to stick to that so simple and straightforward sounding recipe eat less, move more and just do it.

It never worked and will never work for the plain reason that the recipe bypasses the brain and mind, the two most important factors for achieving lasting success.

Again, that's where this book steps in. By explaining how the brain and the mind work and by providing tools and strategies that clearly tell what to do, why to do it, how to do it and where to begin, it will help you to align your actions with your intentions and work consistently toward your goals.

All it requires from you is an open mind as it asks you to take in new information and replace information that may have worked in the past but that no longer serves you.

A great part of this book goes into the working of the brain, part of the central nervous system (CNS), harboring the mind and controlling every function in the body. It is the first responsible for our physical and mental well-being and can be our biggest friend or foe, supporter or opponent. Whatever you achieve or fail to achieve in life, you can largely thank or blame your brain for it.

Of course, we own our brain. It is in our head, it is ours and we therefore have every control over it.

Well, we know that's just theory. Some may be better than others at mastering the processes in their brain but we all have our weak spots, otherwise issues such as lack of willpower, procrastination and stress would never exist.

Your brain is your ultimate gateway to a successful and a fulfilling life, which is why understanding the working of the brain is such an important aspect of this book.

In easy to understand terms it covers how the various parts of our brain function and which buttons to push to create positive results and feelings of reward and joy to replace the negative beliefs and habits in your mind that keep you from achieving your goals.

Not being aware of the processes that occur in your brain and mind and how to organize and use them to your advantage makes it almost impossible to improve health and lose weight.

On the other hand, bringing your brain and mind in line with your intentions will get you every day closer toward your personal health and fitness goals. Also, knowing how to make your brain and mind work for you instead of against will help you with many other aspects of your life.

It is my firm belief as personal fitness trainer, older adult specialist and certified coach practitioner that you will read everything you need to know to put and keep yourself on track toward a better quality of life, for the rest of your life.

In the pages that follow I'll talk about three pillars that together create a solid foundation for achieving and maintaining a healthy lifestyle.

The first pillar, "Mastering Your Life", gives tools and strategies to strengthen and master your willpower and establish a strong and secure self-image.

The second pillar, "Eating for Life", gives extensive information on healthy nutrition and the steps to take to implement healthy eating habits into your lifestyle.

The third pillar, "Moving for Life", covers the ins and outs about safe, efficient, effective and enjoyable exercising and how to make them a natural part of busy week schedule.

To complete the picture, you will read how to combine these three pillars to create a smooth running body, physically as well as mentally, that allows you to create the life you choose to live.

Get what's yours.
To Your Health and Success!

Patrick Streppel
Certified personal fitness trainer and older adult fitness specialist
Certified fitness nutrition coach
Certified coach practitioner

Introduction

Congratulations on purchasing this book!

This book comprises three parts that will take you on a journey toward living a worthwhile and fulfilling healthy lifestyle, "Mastering Your Life", "Eating for Life" and "Moving for Life". They form the reflection of a body and mind that support and stimulate each other in every aspect of your life and throughout your life.

This book is meant for people who have reached a stage in their life where they don't feel good about themselves for reasons of being overweight, lacking strength and energy and an overall suffering health.

It is for those who have come to the conclusion that they have been neglecting their health for too long for reasons such as always putting others' interests first or lacking the time. They know that they still have decades ahead of them filled with possibilities for self-fulfillment but also know that in order to get the best out of those years they need to be in good health.

This book is also for people who have tried to get back in shape several times on their own using various products and programs, failed repeatedly, but still have the will to improve their health and fitness before it is too late.

We all know that regular physical activity and proper nutrition are essential for a healthy body and mind. Fact is that it is for most of us hard to put it all together and keep ourselves on track.

This book explains in a clear and easy to understand format which processes take place in your body when we age and provides you with a workable plan of action to reverse the negative effects of aging and make you achieve your health and fitness goals in a safe, effective, efficient and enjoyable manner.

First an outline of the three parts in this book.

"Mastering Your life", Part One, begins with an overview of the nervous system, how it controls the body's organ systems and explains the role and function of the conscious and subconscious mind. It continues with tools and techniques you can use to begin the process of conditioning how you think, how you feel, what you believe, what you expect and ultimately what you do as it relates to your goals.

"Eating for Life", Part Two, explains the meaning of supportive eating, the effects and benefits of healthy nutrition and how to optimize your food intake during the day to make your body and mind perform at their best.

This part is symbolized by five circles,

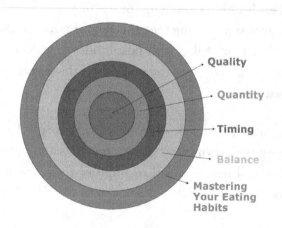

5 Circles Healthy Nutrition

"Quality" is the core of healthy eating habits; knowing which food makes you feel, look and perform better.

"Quantity" is next, knowing when enough is enough and how to prevent overeating.

"Timing" is the third circle, how to plan and strategize eating and drinking throughout the day.

"Balance", the fourth circle, goes into balancing food intake with type and level of physical activity and your personal metabolic blue print.

"Mastering Your Eating Habits" circle encloses the previous four, keeps them consistent with each other and builds upon the tools and techniques of Part One with the purpose to help with implementing healthy eating habits.

At the end of the book you'll find the following five documents that belong to this part:

- Time-Bender Exercise
- The Weekly Meal Plan with Shopping List
- Template Shopping List
- Food and Fluid Journal
- Checklist Achieving and Maintaining a Healthy Weight

"Moving for Life", Part Three, covers everything you need to know for building physical strength and improving flexibility. It contains full body workout routines you can easily vary, together with descriptions and pictures of the exercises. It has also a checklist and a chart to keep track of your results.

This part is also symbolized by five circles;

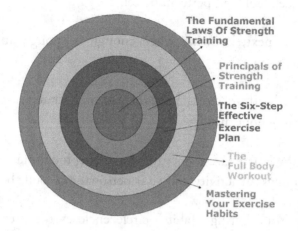

The Fundamental
Laws Of Strength
Training

Principals of
Strength
Training

The Six-Step
Effective
Exercise
Plan

The
Full Body
Workout

Mastering
Your Exercise
Habits

5 circles Safe and Effective Exercising

"Fundamental Laws of a Strength Training" is the first circle and consists of six laws that ensure a safe, effective, efficient and enjoyable training program.

"Principles of Strength Training" is the second circle, builds upon the first circle and encompasses five principles that help you improving your results and achieving your goals.

"The Six-Step Effective Exercise Plan" is the third circle and explains the plan that helps you with setting realistic goals and provides you with a roadmap for achieving those goals.

"The Full Body Workout" is the fourth circle and describes a workout you can do on your own at home or in a gym, with or without weights, activates all areas of the body and that offers suggestions to keep the workouts inspiring and challenging.

"Mastering Your Exercise Habits" is the fifth circle. Similar to the fifth circle of Part Two it encloses the previous four, keeps them consistent with one another and builds upon the tools and techniques of Part One with the purpose to help implementing a safe and effective exercise routine.

Belonging to this part you'll find at the end of this book a checklist for optimizing the results of your training program and a workout journal.

There you have it, three pillars that serve as a foundation for a healthy lifestyle. Know that once you have made yourself familiar with the contents of this book, you'll almost automatically begin to expand what you have learned to other aspects of your life.

So make your start and begin reading. Learn, grow and have fun with it.

Part One

"Mastering Your Life"

After reading the preface and introduction you probably understand why this book, unlike most other books about losing weight and regaining strength and energy, first discusses how the brain and mind work.

Everything begins, ends and begins again in the head, brain and mind.

There's no rocket science, just straight forward information, giving you the insight that forms the foundation for establishing healthy lifestyle habits. The information explains how the brain, the most important part of the nervous system, processes the information it receives from our five senses seeing, hearing, feeling, tasting and smelling, and how you can guide your brain to process the information.

Welcome therefore to the title of this chapter "Mastering Your Life". Once you know how to master the processes in your brain, you'll become the conductor of your life and will be able to live your life the way you choose.

The secret to lasting success is to make the process fun, and that is precisely what happens when you know which buttons to push. Understanding how your brain, mind and body work and how they interact puts you in charge, and this feeling of being in control makes all the difference.

We'll start by looking at the hardware or anatomy of the nervous system, the organ system which controls every function of the human body, making it the first responsible for our physical and mental well-being.

Take your time to read through this information for it will come back when we cover the topics of healthy nutrition and safe and effective exercising in Parts Two and Three.

After reviewing the hardware, it's time to take a look at the software or programming of the mind. Here we arrive at the core of where the magic happens.

The mind houses our conscious and subconscious, the place where we process our thoughts and feelings, where we create our beliefs, habits and expectations, and ultimately our life.

Without aligning the processes that occur in our mind with the goals we pursue, achieving success will be unlikely. That's why 95 to 98 percent of the people who try to improve their health and quality of life through losing weight and regaining strength and energy, for instance, fail repeatedly.

I therefore recommend that you first make yourself familiar with Part One of this book "Mastering Your Life" and then dive into Parts Two and Three, "Eating for Life" and "Moving for Life".

I hope that you'll find it to be a fun and rewarding journey that will change your life for the better, for the rest of your life.

The Anatomy of the Nervous System

The nervous system's role and function is to continuously collect, process and store information about its internal and external states. The system is made of neurons or nerve cells and comprises the central nervous system, consisting of the brain and the spinal cord, and the peripheral nervous system, the vast network of nerves throughout the body, linking to the spinal cord and brain.

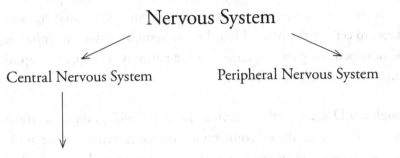

Neurons, see the image below, have three parts, a cell body or nucleus, dendrites or thread like structures surrounding the cell body for incoming signals and axons or nerve fibers, which are meant for outgoing signals and are connected to thousands of other neurons. These axons can vary in length from a millimeter to a meter.

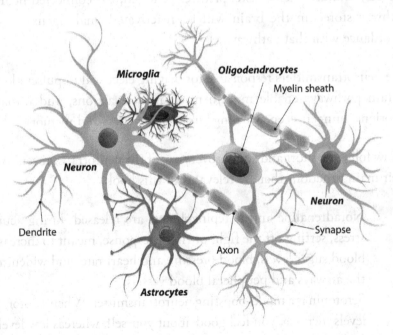

Nerve Cell

The point where the axon of a neuron connects to the dendrite of another neuron is called a synapse. Every time we see, think, feel, imagine or remember something, electrical impulses coming from or going to the brain cause the release of neurotransmitters that transfer messages to cells of the body. These brain chemicals drive the impulses to the next neuron, part of a same specific pathway, at a speed of up to 250 miles or 400 kilometers per hour.

Through our DNA, repeated learning and experiencing, these electrical impulses create a chain of connections between neurons that form a pattern or pathway in the brain tissue. Because each neuron that becomes part of a pathway can become part of other pathways as well, the number of pathways that can be created is virtually limitless. This in turn makes the brain's ability to learn, remember and store information nearly endless.

Every time our mind remembers an experience triggered by words, phrases, sounds, smells, taste, pictures or touch, the connected neural pathway stored in the brain will be reactivated, making us act in accordance with that pathway.

The neurotransmitters responsible for driving electrical impulses along certain pathways enable movement or muscle actions, and initiate emotions, hunger, sleep, learning, arousal, alertness and memory.

Below follows a short and simple overview of the neurotransmitters and their main functions that are relevant for this book.

- Noradrenaline and norepinephrine, are released during acute stress, setting off the fight or flight response, meant to increase blood sugar levels, blood pressure and heart rate, and widening the airways and peripheral blood vessels.
- Serotonin is a mood-boosting neurotransmitter. When serotonin levels increase, you feel good about yourself, whereas low levels make you feel sad, depressed and lonely.

When you're feeling down, thinking back to a past success or about something you feel grateful for promotes the release of serotonin and will make you quickly feel better.

Serotonin also influences hunger. It gives you a satisfied feeling and therefore acts as a natural appetite suppressant. Keep your serotonin levels up and you'll find it easier to lose weight.

The nerve cells in the gut take care of the production of about 80 to 90 percent of this neurotransmitter, which explains its important role in digestion. Other functions of serotonin are regulating the sleep and wake cycle, pain control, arousal and promoting the function of other neurotransmitters.

Drugs such as ecstasy and LSD are known for causing an immense increase in serotonin levels.

- Gamma aminobutyric acid (GABA) is nature's version of valium. It decreases brain activity and produces a calming effect for clear thinking.

- Dopamine influences movement, mood, learning and focus/attention. It drives our motivation to get things done. This neurotransmitter is released in anticipation of a new stimulus.

Dopamine is part of the brain's reward pathway that gives a reward in the form of feeling good for choosing activities that enhances the chance of survival as a species.

Think of activities fundamental to life such as eating, drinking, sex, shelter and the upbringing and caring for offspring. The feel good reward connected to the specific action stimulates someone to remember and repeat the associated action.

An example of dopamine's effect would be buying a DVD that you've been waiting to be released. Dopamine inundates your brain when you feel excited on your way to the store, and drops once you have the DVD in your hands and leave the store.

- Endorphins work like morphine. The name endorphin is a combination of endogenous morphine. Endogenous means produced within the body. Endorphins block pain, for instance during natural childbirth, but are also responsible for feelings of bliss and pleasure.

Endorphins take over where dopamine ends. Using the example about purchasing the DVD; endorphins are responsible for the feeling of pleasure when you watch the film. Another example is the feeling of satisfaction when having sex or eating a scrumptious meal.

- Anandamide, also known as the bliss compound blocks feelings of pain and depression. A deficiency of this neurotransmitter leads to stress and anxiety. Although endorphins are often associated with the bliss-like feeling endurance runners call a runners high, recent studies have shown that anandamide is probably more responsible for this effect than endorphins. The reason is that endorphins can't cross the blood-brain barrier, whereas anandamide can.

The Difference between Hormones and Neurotransmitters

Neurotransmitters send messages to cells of the body and so do hormones.

The difference between the two is the release mechanisms. Neurons produce neurotransmitters, which use the nervous system as a transmission mechanism, whereas the endocrine glands produce hormones, which use the blood stream as a transmission mechanism.

Due to the nature of the mechanisms, neurotransmitters act extremely fast whereas hormones act more slowly and can last from seconds to days.

Part One of the Central Nervous System, The Brain

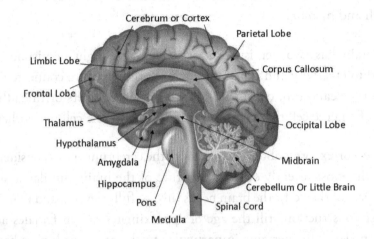

Brain

The human brain consists of about 86 billion neurons or nerve cells, each capable of making 10,000 connections. The brain is 2 percent of the body's weight, consumes 20 to 30 percent of the daily calorie intake and consists in fact of three brains; the cortex, the limbic brain and the reptilian brain.

The Cerebrum or Cortex

The first brain is the cerebrum, or cortex, and is the largest of the three. It is linked to higher brain functions such as thought and action. It has four sections, called lobes, each with specific functions, such as the following:

Frontal lobe: problem solving, logic, intellect, reasoning, planning, movement and parts of speech

Parietal lobe: movement, recognition and orientation

Occipital lobe: vision

Temporal lobe (behind the temples, not visible on the image): hearing, speech and memory

The brain has two hemispheres or halves. The right hemisphere is linked to creativity and the left to logic. Both halves are connected by the corpus callosum, consisting of axons or nerve fibers or threadlike parts of a nerve cell that transport impulses form one cell to another.

The neocortex forms about 90 percent of the cerebrum and is considered to be the most recently evolved structure of the brain. Similar to any other part of the body, the brain needs time to fully develop and remains "under construction" till the age of approximately 25 in females and 28 in males. This pertains in particular to the areas for higher brain functions such as the neocortex where new tissue and connections are continuously added.

As an a-side line, this is why you can't really blame adolescents for their sometimes problem causing behavior, as the development of the parts of their brain connected to emotions, planning and decision making takes time.

The Limbic Brain

The second brain is the limbic, mammalian or emotional brain located below the cerebrum or cortex. It is the area of the brain that combines higher mental functions with primitive emotions and consists of four major parts.

The first part is the thalamus where almost all sensory information enters and is sent forth to the overlying cortex.

The second part is the hypothalamus, responsible for a number of functions such as controlling the pituitary gland or master gland. This gland regulates the thyroid gland which produces thyroxine and the adrenals that produce cortisol.

Other functions of the hypothalamus are regulating emotions, thirst, hunger, sleep/wake rhythms and the autonomic nervous system explained below.

The hypothalamus is also important for maintaining homeostasis, the state of balance in the body where all body functions occur smoothly and the demand for energy matches with the supply of energy.

Third part is the amygdala which comprises two clusters of nerve cells with the shape of almonds. They are involved in preparing the body for the fight and flight response and in storing of information, particularly those related to emergencies and emotional events. They also play a role in the development of extreme fear and storing long-term memories.

The fourth major part of the limbic brain is the hippocampus, important for learning, converting short term memory to long term memory and for registering information about the environment and the events we experience, real or imagined.

The amount of information that can be stored in the hippocampus is enormous. Studies have shown that London taxi drivers have an enlarged hippocampus due to spending years on committing the numerous streets to memory.

The hippocampus is very vulnerable to continuous stress. Stress and the related stress hormone cortisol can damage neurons which in turn can cause the hippocampus to shrink.

The Reptilian Brain

The third brain is the reptilian brain consisting of the cerebellum and the brainstem. The brainstem in turn consists of the midbrain, pons and medulla.

The cerebellum, also known as little brain and hindbrain, is associated with posture, balance and coordination of movement.

The brainstem regulates basic functions such as heartbeat, breathing, body temperature and blood pressure.

The reptilian brain is seen from an evolutionary viewpoint the oldest and most powerful of the three brains. It is an instinctive, primitive brain all reptiles, mammals and humans are equipped with.

Survival is the number one job of our brain and in particular of the reptilian brain. Because the reptilian brain works instinctively, we don't even need to think before we act to protect ourselves when we feel in danger or injured.

Examples of instinctive responses of the reptilian brain are attack or run, aggression, fear, anger, revenge, reproduction and territorial behavior.

Part Two of The Central Nervous System, The Spinal Cord

The second part of the central nervous system, the spinal cord, resides within the vertebral column. The main tasks of the vertebral column are providing stability and flexibility for movement, transmitting body weight and protecting the spinal cord.

The spinal cord is about 45 centimeters or 18 inches long in men and 43 centimeters or 17 inches long in women, runs from the base of the skull to the lower back and connects the brain through 31 pairs of spinal nerves with the peripheral nervous system.

The two functions of the spinal cord are providing a two way street for signals coming from and going to the brain and handling reflexes. To avoid delay, not the brain but the spinal cord regulates reflex actions. The brain analyzes and processes the event after the reflex.

The Peripheral Nervous System

The peripheral nervous system, see the image below, is the vast network of nerves throughout the body that carries information from within and outside the body to the spinal cord and brain and carries commands from the brain via the spinal cord to all parts of the body.

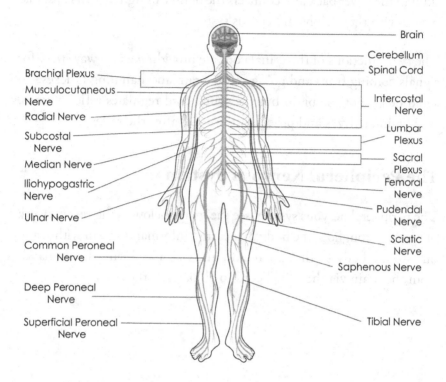

- Brain
- Cerebellum
- Spinal Cord
- Intercostal Nerve
- Lumbar Plexus
- Sacral Plexus
- Femoral Nerve
- Pudendal Nerve
- Sciatic Nerve
- Saphenous Nerve
- Tibial Nerve

Brachial Plexus
Musculocutaneous Nerve
Radial Nerve
Subcostal Nerve
Median Nerve
Iliohypogastric Nerve
Ulnar Nerve
Common Peroneal Nerve
Deep Peroneal Nerve
Superficial Peroneal Nerve

NERVOUS SYSTEM

The peripheral nervous system divides into the somatic nervous system controlling the *voluntary* skeletal muscle contractions and the autonomic nervous system controlling the *involuntary* muscle contractions of blood vessels, smooth muscles, which are muscles that surround or are part of internal organs, cardiac muscles and the internal organs that make up the digestive system. The diagram below summarizes how the peripheral nervous system is organized.

Peripheral Nervous System

Autonomic Nervous System
(involuntary muscle contractions)

Somatic Nervous System
(voluntary muscle contractions)

Sympathetic Nervous System

Parasympathetic Nervous System

The autonomic nervous system regulates the body's unconscious actions and consists of the sympathetic and the parasympathetic nervous system. They function in opposition to each other and work on the smooth muscles of the internal organs. When one system excites, the other inhibits.

It is the hypothalamus, part of the limbic brain that controls the autonomic nervous system.

Other names for parasympathetic nervous system are the rest and digest system or the feed and breed system. When this system dominates, the body is in a relaxed state where digestion and assimilation, healing, recovering and building of new body tissue can occur.

When the sympathetic nervous system dominates, the body is in a state of survival, also known as fight or flight. The secretion of stress hormones such as adrenaline and cortisol directs blood from the gut section to the arms and legs for running or fighting and to the brain for fast thinking. Blood vessels and airways widen, heart rate increases and blood pressure raises.

How the Automatic Nervous System Influences our Metabolism

Translated to our daily life it means that our mental state, relaxed, stressed or somewhere in between, determines which of the two systems dominates and whether the metabolic processes that occur in our body are either anabolic or catabolic.

Metabolism is the total of chemical processes that occur in the body necessary for growth, repair and maintenance of body tissue, to produce energy and to eliminate waste.

When in an anabolic state, also known as condensation, the body is in a state of growth, meaning that it is binding nutrients from food or components in the body for growth, repair and maintenance. It is in this state that the parasympathetic nervous system dominates.

When shifted into a catabolic state, also known as hydrolysis, the body is breaking down nutrients from food or components in the body to produce energy. In this state the sympathetic nervous system dominates.

It makes sense that our mental state has a big impact on the metabolic processes in our body when we eat, drink or workout.

Not being aware of the impact of these two conditions on the processes of digestion and assimilation is one of the main reasons many people feel disappointed when they don't see the reward for their hard work in the form of weight loss and strength gain.

Let's have a closer look at the effects on the body when we are mentally stressed in relation to the two examples just mentioned, losing weight and gaining strength.

Stress, real or imagined, minor or major, shifts the body into survival mode, activates the sympathetic nervous system and prepares the body for fighting or running and hiding. The adrenal glands and the pancreas secrete hormones into the blood stream causing an instant release of all available energy. At the same time, heart rate and breathing quicken, blood pressure increases, blood vessels and airways widen and blood flow moves from the midsection of the body to the head for quick thinking and to the arms and legs for fighting or running and hiding.

Depending on the level, stress reduces the activity of body functions that don't play a crucial role in dealing with the perceived threat to a minimum. Examples are digestion, assimilation, healing and recovery.

Bottom line is that regardless of the quality of your exercise program and of how healthy and balanced you eat, if done in a stressed state, not much can be expected from efforts geared to losing weight and regaining strength and energy.

Maintaining a state of relaxation obviously results in the opposite effects. When we feel relaxed the parasympathetic nervous system dominates and body functions linked to anabolism such as digestion, assimilation, healing and recovery occur easily. Being in this state opens the doors to achieving health and fitness goals such as weight loss and strength building.

Parts Two and Three go further into the effects of stress on eating, drinking and exercising.

This brings us to the question how to recognize and deal with stress. Before we can answer this question, we'll need to go into the role and function of the conscious and subconscious mind or the software of the brain as they relate to stress, memory and behavior.

The Conscious and The Subconscious Mind

Previously we covered the hardware of the brain consisting of three main sections, the cortex, the limbic brain and the reptilian brain.

The subconscious and conscious mind represent the software or programming of the brain. The limbic system is the home of the subconscious mind, and the front part of the cortex or prefrontal cortex is the home of the conscious mind.

The subconscious mind regulates mental processes such as emotions, arousal and memory formation. It also manages our automatic responses and is the place where we store our beliefs, expectations, values, attitudes and habits.

The conscious mind is the thinking part of the mind linked to awareness, problem solving, logic, intellect, reasoning, justifying, planning, negotiating, movement, parts of speech, willpower and short- and mid-term memory.

The conscious mind and subconscious mind live in close relationship and ideally interact with each other in harmony. However, understanding their differences in characteristics, this is not always the case.

The limbic brain, home of the subconscious mind, is the strongest. It can stimulate the performance of the prefrontal cortex, home of the conscious mind, through the release of the feel good hormone dopamine by the hypothalamus, or it can override and shut down the processes in the prefrontal cortex by signaling the adrenal glands to release the stress hormone cortisol when activating the fight or flight response.

The subconscious mind represents the hot area of the brain and can act emotionally and impulsively, whereas the conscious mind represents the cool area that acts well behaved, considerate and analytic.

Another important difference is that the subconscious mind works day and night without interruption, whereas the conscious mind only comes into action when we consciously engage ourselves to a task. This means that if we don't keep our conscious mind alert and active, our subconscious mind will be in charge of our behavior.

Involved in emotions, memory formation and long term memories, the limbic brain automatically takes in all the information that passes the reticular activating system (RAS), a filtering network that lets data through following three criteria.

The first criterion is that the information is important for survival. Examples are waking up in the middle of the night because of a strange sound or the sound of crying child. The second reaction in particular is related to new moms who tend to wake up and jump out of bed on the first cry of their child.

The second criterion is that the information is new, unfamiliar or different. An example is immediately noticing a new object in a room. The reason you don't notice it any more after a few weeks is that it has become familiar.

The last of the three criteria is that the information has a high emotional content. The more an experience is charged with emotion, the easier it becomes part of your memory. You don't remember every trip to work or school but you will remember the one you witnessed a serious car accident.

The limbic brain has no sense of time and doesn't reason or asks questions. It only takes in and processes the data that pass the RAS filter from the moment we are born.

Even though the RAS filter prevents too much information from entering the brain, it still is a very basic filter. It is the job of the rational conscious mind to play the role of gate keeper. Being a much more selective filter, the conscious mind analyzes and questions the incoming information and only accepts what it, subjectively, recognizes as safe, familiar and known.

You can compare the relationship between the subconscious and the conscious mind to a radio telescope with connected data bank and an operator, where the radio telescope represents the five senses seeing, hearing, feeling, smelling and tasting, the connected databank the subconscious mind and the operator the conscious mind.

Without analyzing and filtering the incoming data, the data just keep coming in. It is the work of the operator to analyze the incoming data and to filter out the information of no value.

It makes sense that we can get into trouble when we neglect or forget to remain alert and allow information to enter our brain and influence our behavior.

Describing how commercials work is a good example. Marketers put a lot of effort in finding ways to bypass the consumer's conscious mind and directly access their subconscious mind where their marketing message can hit the consumer's bliss point, the point where the resistance is the lowest and sets off the biggest amount of craving.

Through using the optimal combination of words, tone, pictures, colors and repetition, marketers try to set off a feel good response in our brain we can't resist. The hour of the day we are presented with commercials also plays an important role. As an example, late night commercials are broadcasted late night because that is for most of us the part of the day that our energy levels and consequently the resistance of our conscious mind are at their lowest.

And so we grab our credit card and buy the product.

Good for you if using your common sense is what you normally do, for that enables you to reconsider your purchase the next morning when you feel refreshed and energized.

If you don't use your conscious mind, you rob yourself from your free will and make yourself vulnerable for influences whose interests are not necessarily yours.

Understanding the role and function of the conscious mind makes you realize how vulnerable you were during the first two decades of your life. The fact that the prefrontal cortex takes so long to mature greatly influences how we develop from childhood to adulthood with regard to our thoughts, feelings, believes, expectations and habits.

From the moment we arrive on this planet, our mind immediately begins to passively take in and record all the information it receives via its senses, similar to a film that records an image coming through the lens of a camera.

As mentioned, the limbic brain doesn't judge any of this information. It doesn't have any idea of time and place, lives in the present, doesn't have a will of its own and can't tell the difference between real or imagined. It just takes in the information that has passed the RAS filter, accepts it as true and stores everything.

The vulnerability of children underlines the enormous responsibility adults have when interacting with them. All experiences, good or bad, can become ingrained in an instant, especially those that are emotionally charged, and can play an important role during the rest of life.

The subconscious mind automatically compares events, real or imagined, with the stored information from previous events and responds with automatic reactions that match with the event.

About 95 percent of our behavior is habit and we are only aware of 10 to 15 percent. Think of an ice berg of which you can see only 10 to 15 percent because the rest is under water. This is an asset of high value since it allows us to move smoothly and quickly from one event to the other without having to spend time and energy on reinventing the wheel every time. Just think of how awkward it would be if you had to learn every time again how to use a phone.

A wide range of triggers can set off an automatic reaction from the subconscious mind. Examples are sounds, words, phrases, sentences, smells, touch and tastes. In other words, anything that comes to us through one or more of our five senses, seeing, hearing, feeling, tasting and smelling can lead to physical and/or emotional reactions that are connected to specific feelings, beliefs, expectations and habits.

In many situations these automatic reactions are useful for quickly recalling personal experiences like a vacation, graduations, family gatherings etcetera. Unfortunately these automatic reactions can also be in our way when they result in unsupportive habits and behavior such as emotional eating, nail biting or nervousness before giving a public performance.

Both the conscious and the subconscious mind have their strengths and advantages. The subconscious mind can contribute to a spontaneous and vivid personality and is famous for the light bulb moments. The quality of the conscious mind is to create rest and build in a pause between the stimulus from one or more of the five senses and the reaction from the subconscious mind.

This last feature is helpful to make you think twice before you come with a reaction. Think of an adult with a fully developed conscious mind who realizes just in time that it is best to say nothing in a particular situation, whereas a child or an adolescent with a not yet fully developed conscious mind directly reacts with a spontaneous inappropriate comment.

This doesn't mean that we always have to be so happy with our conscious mind. Problem is that it sometimes finds it difficult to make up its mind, which can result in endless doubting, evaluating, analyzing, rationalizing and justifying, which in turn can lead to, for instance, procrastinating.

And when the conscious mind finally has made up its mind, it is likely that it has built its decision of what is right or wrong, possible or impossible, realistic or unrealistic, on the secure and familiar beliefs and habits stored in the subconscious mind.

It makes sense that for the purpose of creating a harmonious relationship the conscious and subconscious mind can do with some guidance.

This guidance can obviously only come from one person, you.

By consciously applying the strength and the power of the conscious mind wisely, you can take the decisions that are in alignment with your goals in life.

Many people are unaware of the effect information coming through their senses has on their thoughts and feelings, how they create beliefs and expectations and eventually determine their habits,

Since they also don't realize that they can play a leading role in the process of forming beliefs and expectations, they live on autopilot and behave in accordance with how the subconscious mind has become programmed over the years.

Living on autopilot is the opposite of living mindfully. Living on autopilot means one is not really aware of what is going on, is not in the moment, is not present. It is the cause of near all of our suffering.

Creating awareness about the processes in our mind and influencing them to our advantage is a first condition for living mindfully. Mindfulness promotes health and well-being and begins with understanding how beliefs, expectations and habits take shape as a result of thoughts and feelings.

How Memories, Beliefs, Habits and Expectations Take Shape and Cling To You

Remember that the components that form the subconscious mind are the hippocampus and the amygdala.

Information coming from the reticular activating system (RAS) goes first to the amygdala where it is given an emotional value before it is passed on to the hippocampus. The latter compares the data with those already stored as long-term memory and sends then them via the thalamus to the cortex for evaluation after which the data become part of the long-term memory.

The type of memory that is stored in the hippocampus is autobiographical, holding a journal of the events you were part of. The information it registers comprises day and hour of the event, the environment, who and what else was there and what emotions were involved.

When you think back to such an event, for instance your wedding or that of a close relative, you can see yourself acting in these moments and recall details such as clothing, scents, sounds and facial expressions.

Parts of the memories such as these will be stored in other parts of the brain as well, but it is through the hippocampus that they remain linked to one another. The more emotionally charged these events, the better you will be able to recall them later.

Every time your mind is triggered through what you hear, see, smell, feel, taste or think, associations will appear in your mind related to the event that created the memory.

The events we are part of not only produce memories but also thoughts and feelings that in turn lead to beliefs, expectations and habits.

When the brain receives information through one or more of our senses, it searches its data bank, pulls up the map with information it recognizes as similar to the event and sets off an automatic reaction that is congruent with the information organized and stored in that particular map in your brain.

Remember that 95 percent of our days are filled with automatic reactions in the form of beliefs and expectations that lead to decisions, choices, behavior and habits.

The word habit originally means garment. Reasons we wear garments or clothes are because we like them and they protect and fit us. But no matter how much we like them, there comes a time we want to dispose of them and look for clothes that suit us better.

Beliefs, habits and expectations that no longer suit us should get the same treatment.

This may sound like a simple thing to do but not for most people. Already identifying unsupportive thoughts, beliefs and expectations can be hard, changing them even harder.

The purpose of the first part of this book is helping you solving this puzzle.

Before going into this, we need to go over the role and function of the amygdala, the other half of the subconscious mind.

Similar to the hippocampus, the amygdala is programmed to automatically react to stimuli. The difference is that the amygdala is specialized in stress reactions, setting off a surge to fight, to flight or to freeze.

In response to an event that causes a stress reaction, the hypothalamus, also part of the limbic brain, immediately stimulates the secretion of the associated stress hormones cortisol and adrenaline leading to the physical responses we covered before.

Preparing and charging the body for dealing with the perceived threat or emergency requires a follow-up in the form of physical activity to get the pressure of the kettle and release the abundance of energy.

In the absence of physical activity like running or fighting, the follow-up appears in the form of actions such as pacing up and down a room, pawing the ground, heavy breathing, sweating, yelling, and so on. It takes about 20 to 60 minutes to recover from a stress situation.

In case stress responses have a milder form, the external effects may not or hardly be noticeable but internally the effects are undeniable and take form through partly inhibiting body functions that have no role in dealing with the emergency. Examples of these body functions are digestion, assimilation, recovery and healing.

Stress can take shape in many different ways and its symptoms can come from problems with work, relationships, money, family, health, sexuality or purpose in life. The more and the longer we deal with stressful situations, the more they become ingrained and the stronger the symptoms are felt every time the events occur.

These symptoms come in four varieties, emotional, physical, behavioral and cognitive.

Examples of emotional symptoms are feeling down, sad and depressed, irritated, agitated, overwhelmed, lonely and/or alone and moody.

Examples of physical symptoms are gaining weight or not able to lose weight, digestive problems, frequent colds, no libido, nervousness, pressure on chest and elevated heart rate, discomforts and pains, nausea and dizziness.

Examples of behavioral symptoms are binge eating, not eating or less than normal, wishing to be left alone, avoiding responsibilities, procrastinating, trying to destress with alcohol, drugs/medication and smoking, taking up nervous habits, not sleeping well or staying in bed too long.

Examples of cognitive symptoms are focusing on negatives, constantly worrying, difficulty with concentrating, forgetting things, jumpy mind, expecting the worst and being judgmental.

We are all subject to stress now and then and there is nothing wrong with that. Important in the first place is how we perceive stress and how we deal with it.

Giving a positive twist to stress can bring us in a state of excitement and alertness, enabling us to deal with important situations such as giving a speech, pushing ourselves when exercising or competing against others.

The story becomes different when stress has a negative load and leads to symptoms as mentioned above. The purpose of stress reactions is to deal with situations that only last for a short while and not for situations that last long, as is the case in the life of so many people nowadays.

When talking about stress we are quick to say that stress may be a problem to others, but not to us, that we are fine and that we don't recognize ourselves in the symptoms. One reason we tend to react like this is that we fear that others will see us as weak and not capable to deal with stressful situations.

Another reason may be that even though we recognize the feeling of stress, we don't know what to do about it and therefore rather ignore than address it.

Recognizing the presence of stress in our life can also be a source of stress in itself as it tells us that we have to develop or improve our strengths and/or skills to deal with stress. This not only drives us out of our comfort zone, but also demands our time and continuous effort, which doesn't sound appealing considering our overloaded agenda.

On the other hand, when we realize that living in stress equals living in survival and know how stress affects our health, we must understand that we need to bring up the courage to acknowledge its existence and take action to reduce or eliminate what causes the stress.

The Creation of the Unique Picture of Your "Self"

What the automatic reactions of the hippocampus and the amygdala have in common is that some help us to move closer toward our goals, whereas others do the exact opposite.

Identifying unsupportive automatic reactions in the form of beliefs, habits and expectations is not always easy since you may not even know that you have them. A simple example would be asking someone why he is doing something in a certain way and getting a response in return sounding like: "I don't know, this is just how I always do it".

Remember that it takes around 25 years for the prefrontal cortex to mature before the conscious mind can fully take up its role as gate keeper and analyze what comes in, goes out and what is stored. And even when it has become fully developed, it may not always be alert.

The problem is that as long as we don't develop and train our conscious mind and apply it by consistently questioning our beliefs and expectations, our subconscious mind will always perceive these beliefs and expectations as the objective truth and force us to act accordingly whether we like it or not.

It is what makes people say "This is the way I am" or "This is who I am and what I am" and "You can't teach an old dog new tricks".

I recall meeting with a woman who was in her fifties and significantly overweight. She had trouble with moving around and walking up the stairs was a real challenge. She mentioned some health problems and uttered frequently statements such as "I don't do that anymore", "I can't do that", "I am too old for that" and "that is not good for me."

Asking her if she had ever considered adjusting her lifestyle so that she could lose some weight and improve her overall health, she told me that her current weight must be her right weight because she never ate much and when she did, only ate healthy food. She also knew that she was active enough because she went out for a walk with her dog at least twice a day.

She acknowledged that her health was not optimal but that was because her mother had the same health issues and that she therefore must have inherited them. For the rest it was simply a fact of growing older, a fact of life that when you're in your fifties, you can't do the things anymore you were used to do when you were in your thirties.

This story is not unique. In my conversations with men and women who have entered their second part of life I hear these types of stories more often than not.

These stories are often the result of not understanding the changes that occur in the body during the various phases in life, not understanding the mental processes that are responsible for the forming of beliefs and expectations, and not knowing or believing that everybody has the ability to take charge and control these processes.

Whatever our subconscious mind perceives as the objective truth will always form the basis for what we think is possible, our comfort-zone and how we perceive ourselves, our self-image.

The woman I had the conversation with accepted life as it came to her and had no idea that her beliefs and expectations had created the life she was going through and that she could give her life another direction by changing those beliefs and expectations.

Awareness is the first necessary condition for change. The awareness that something is missing in life sets off the necessary urge for change. Fact is however that awareness alone isn't enough to make a change in our life. Numerous people live with the awareness something is missing but never get further than feeling frustrated and angry because they are unable to fill the void in their life or make lasting changes.

Understanding the working of our brain and mind is the second necessary condition for change. Without this it is impossible to discover that it is our mind that created the beliefs we perceive as the objective truth and is responsible for the life we are experiencing.

The word "discover" I used in the previous sentence is the key to change. Change comes from within. Only by discovering yourself how your mind functions you can become aware that you have full control over the processes that create beliefs and expectations.

What automatically follows is that you'll begin to influence those processes and help your subconscious mind with replacing the beliefs and expectations that are holding you back from living the life you want.

Tools and techniques in this book will help you with this.

You can read a million quotes about healthy living, but if you only accept those wise words with your conscious mind and not with your subconscious mind, you will never truly accept them and will never be able to change.

When people feel a void in their life they tend to look for solutions outside themselves. The last place they look is inside their own mind because their objective truth tells them that the problem can't be their objective truth.

Learn how your brain and mind work and you'll discover the silliness of your objective truth, how it filled itself with self-imposed limitations and created your self-image and comfort-zone, both reflecting what you think is possible.

As with any device, you have to understand how it works. If you do, you feel happy. If you don't you feel frustrated. The solution is in fact simple; find the manual, read it, discover which buttons you need to push and enjoy the ride.

The process of learning to understand how your brain and mind work takes time because of the numerous different experiences you go through every day. What you will notice quickly is that you begin to observe and reflect upon your feelings and thoughts and become the spectator of your life.

The biggest discovery from this is that you'll realize that you *are* not your self-image, you *are* not your thoughts, you *are* not your feelings, you *are* not your beliefs, you *are* not your habits; you *have* them and therefore, you can change them.

Like a coat rack holding coats, hats and shawls, you're holding beliefs etcetera that ultimately determine what your self-image looks like. The big difference between you and a coat rack is that you have the ability to decide which beliefs you want to hold on to and which you want to dispose of.

Changing your self-image is possible. It is not set in stone. Once you understand the processes that create your self-image, you have the ability to modify these processes in a manner that they support positive change and strengthen your self-image.

With changing and strengthening your self-image, your comfort zone will change and expand and subsequently your actions and what you believe is possible. Opportunities and possibilities never considered realistic before come within reach and spark a chain of events that are life changing.

Before changing unsupportive habits, it is important to concentrate on improving your self-image. Trying to change a habit such as smoking or overeating without first improving your self-image will probably result in being pulled back into your old habits quickly since these habits are consistent with the self-image still in place.

To build out the metaphor of the coat rack a bit more; if a coat rack is not standing on an even surface or is not properly attached to a wall, it will never be able to do its job right. Solving this problem by giving the coat rack a solid ground or attachment should therefore be the first step to take.

Improving your self-image automatically creates room for changing unwanted habits. Reason for this is that your self-image encompasses your entire comfort zone, from the core to its outside boundaries, whereas habits and beliefs are just expressions of your self-image and stay within and near the boundaries of the comfort zone.

Just imagine how much easier it will be to establish and maintain supportive habits such as healthy eating and regular exercising when you have a self-image that allows you to feel secure and proud about yourself every day. Living a healthy life style will then almost automatically ensue from that positive self-image.

This is again why this book begins with explaining the processes in your brain and mind that are responsible for what you believe and expect in life and that in turn determine your self-image and how you behave every day.

Following the route of strengthening your self-image first allows you to work from the inside out instead of imposing new habits on yourself, no matter how healthy and wise, which are not consistent with your self-image. Keep in mind that whatever is not aligned with your self-image is something you cannot really believe in and therefore can't hold on to.

The hippocampus, the place for creating long-term memories is the area in your brain where you want to instill an image of yourself that supports you in living the life you choose.

As mentioned before, the hippocampus is part of the limbic brain, the part of the brain that accepts information without judging or reasoning. It doesn't have any idea of time and place, lives in the present, doesn't have a will of its own, and can't tell the difference between real or imagined.

Bottom line is that the human brain is a big bio-computer. You can teach it anything, good or bad. The fact that we arrived on this planet with a clean and empty mind is why we can grow up in any culture, learn any language, become any type of person with any type of profession, all forming our self-image and comfort-zone.

Bombard this bio-computer with messages such as I'm a failure, my life is a mess, I've always had bad luck, I'm just not good at learning new things, and guess what comes out? How would you feel, think, believe and see yourself? The answer is obvious.

It is really that simple. And the beauty of this system is that it works the other way to. Suppose you would say to yourself things like I can do that, I feel happy and secure, I love my life, I can learn how to play a musical instrument, I can and I will find time to do what's good for both my body and mind. Imagine how that would feel and how that would influence what you believe and how you see yourself.

This quote from Buddha reflects it in a few words.

"The mind is everything. What you think you become."

No rocket science here, this is how it works. The sad truth is that most people tolerate negative thoughts, feelings and beliefs in their mind that eventually dictate what their self-image and consequently their comfort-zone and life looks like.

There is nothing wrong with people who have a negative self-image. They only learned the wrong things. As I just mentioned, we *are* not our self-image, we *are* not our thoughts, we *are* not our feelings, we *are* not our beliefs, we *are* not our habits. We *have* them and therefore we can change them.

Your Life and Your Free Will

If you feel that your self-image and where you are in life doesn't reflect your intentions, you may question the status of your free will.

Apparently, at some point in your life thoughts and feelings that were not consistent with your intentions in life managed to find a place in your mind. What happened since is that they became the foundation for your expectations and habits, and that they are now preventing you from moving your life in the direction you desire.

In short, something in your mind is interfering with your free will and is evidently stronger.

It is my conviction and experience that no matter your age, gender, physical abilities and current level of health and fitness, we are always capable of change and growth. We must be, for if we're not we're standing still, which equals moving backwards.

The consequence of moving backwards is that we're looking at a shrinking comfort zone that offers every day a bit less of life than the day before.

We deserve better, much better. And it is good to know that we have science at our side. What the science of neuroplasticity tells us is that our brain is not as unchangeable as a piece of rock but as pliable as a piece of plastic. Whether you are a junior or an older adult, you can teach your brain new beliefs, thoughts and habits, replace those that don't support you and manage impulses that go against your intentions.

The saying you can't teach old dogs new tricks couldn't be further from the truth. The process of changing, learning and developing never ends. You are the architect and conductor of your brain. Sculpt it and use it anyway you want. The only thing needed is an open mind and a willingness to learn for the benefit of yourself, your loved ones and humankind as a whole.

Having a willingness to change and grow equals caring for and respecting yourself and forms the basis for doing the same to others and being a good example.

The opposite is also true. If there is no urge within you to change and grow, it means that you don't care about yourself and don't respect yourself. What you don't possess is impossible to give and teach others.

The most important person in your life is you. You can argue that you live for your spouse, your children or any other person, and that you see them as more important but if you don't look after yourself in the first place, what good can you be to them?

I'm not saying that you need to be in perfect health and shape; you just need to be human, complete with all your imperfections. Essential is that you commit yourself to living a healthy life style to the best of your abilities.

Change is the outcome from learning and comprises three steps. First, being aware something is missing in life, second, a desire and decision to change and fill the emptiness, and third actually taking the steps to make the change.

People often wonder about their purpose in life. If there is one thing that can be considered as a first condition for any purpose, it is good health. Everything in life depends on it and it therefore really doesn't make much sense if achieving and maintaining good health is not the first goal you should strive toward.

Pursuing a healthy lifestyle enables you to get the best out of life for yourself and to help your loved ones to get the best out of their life. More than that, you encourage others to follow your example.

On the other hand, denying yourself the benefits of a healthy lifestyle limits the possibilities in life for yourself and others and puts you at risk for becoming a burden on the life of others and, considering the ever growing health care costs, on society as a whole.

People with good health in general have a positive view of life and run into opportunities they otherwise would have missed. Their often active life style serves as a motor for a series of events that lead them to people and places that provide them with possibilities for developing a fulfilling and rewarding purpose.

And of course, this not only benefits them but also the people they live and meet with.

Every person is different and arrives on this planet with nothing more than his or her unique talents and leaves with nothing. It is one's purpose to discover and use one's unique talents to make a positive difference in the life of others.

Our greatest asset for using our free will is our conscious mind in our prefrontal cortex. Although present in all mammals, the prefrontal cortex is most developed and complex in humans.

If we consciously engage our conscious mind we can express our free will and find our purpose in life. If we don't, we let external forces take over whose interests may not be the same as ours.

With external forces I'm mainly referring to the convenience industry, consisting of the food, pharmaceutical and entertainment industries. With their focus on revenue and market share, they depend on large numbers of consumers with same preferences and same predictable behaviors.

Honoring the diversity in humankind and recognizing the uniqueness of every individual is not in their interest. The limited range of products and services they offer is nothing compared to the enormous potential of variety people carry within them. In order to protect their revenue and market share they first need to overrule the creative mechanisms present in the brain of every human and then overload them with messages that are consistent with the companies' interests.

The proof of the discrepancy between the goals of the convenience industry and that of people can be witnessed all around us. The number of people, adults and children, that are overweight, depressed and suffering from the deadly chronic welfare diseases that hardly occurred a century ago is astounding and increasing every year.

Fact is that the majority of these people will never be able to break free from their devastating lifestyle. They mindlessly accept the repetitive messages from the convenience industry as true and react with behavior and habits that are consistent with that truth, not realizing that their behavior and habits moves them away from the happiness they really desire.

Some people know that their impaired well-being is a result of their lifestyle but either don't care or find it impossible or simply too much trouble to choose for a healthier lifestyle. They often justify their way of living by convincing themselves that it is not yet that bad, that their friends do the same, that the food actually tastes and looks good and that because the food is not forbidden by the government it must be good.

The list with excuses and justifications coming from what I call mind games continuous as long as needed to silence the undercurrent that tries to tell them that they know better.

The people I am holding high are those who keep trying to change their life for the better despite all their previous unsuccessful attempts to break free from the habits that make it impossible to live the life they desire.

It is to these people I say that they have a free will and that they can regain the control over their life. Through applying the qualities of the conscious mind one can make the choices that are consistent with one's goals in life. The techniques explained and described in this book help with developing and training the conscious mind.

Getting Back In Charge with The Power of The Conscious Mind

It is through engaging our conscious mind that we have the ability to replace negative ingrained automatic patterns of thoughts, beliefs, habits and expectations.

This may sound like a profound and far away ideal for you at this stage but it is less complicated than it sounds. Consciously or unconsciously you developed your self-image through experiences in the past. You can change it by the same method.

The prefrontal cortex that harbors the conscious mind provides us with the ability to take charge and, like a conductor in front of an orchestra, grab the conductor's stick and bring harmony in the music that is coming from the orchestra represented by the subconscious mind.

To expand this picture a bit, imagine members of an orchestra who receive a music sheet and decide to immediately begin playing, similar to the subconscious mind that instantly reacts when it receives a stimulus via one or more of the senses.

The music coming from the orchestra will most likely sound chaotic and will continue to do so until a conductor arrives with his conductor's stick and takes control. Not right away, but after some practice each member of the orchestra knows what to do and the orchestra will begin to produce music worth listening to.

Whereas the subconscious mind immediately and automatically reacts to every stimulus, the prefrontal cortex has the ability to build in a short pause between the stimulus and the reaction of the subconscious mind. This short pause, which can take less than a second, is long enough to oversee the options and to choose for the best response.

This is where the neurotransmitter gamma aminobutyric acid (GABA) plays a key role. Through its calming effect this neurotransmitter makes it easier for brain cells to communicate with each other and make better decisions.

Like a conductor who takes charge and steps in front of the orchestra to bring structure and alignment in the orchestra's performance we have the ability to use our conscious mind wisely, bring structure and alignment in the impulsive reactions coming from the subconscious mind and consider the best response.

Be careful here, for what is the best response? Realize that the quality of the response of our conscious mind entirely depends on how well we perform our role as conductor.

Although the conscious mind is linked to qualities such as logic, intellect, reasoning, planning and negotiating, its responses can easily become influenced by beliefs, expectations and values stored in the subconscious mind.

It fully depends on the strengths and skills of our conscious mind how well we are able to understand the true value of the reactions coming from the subconscious mind and consider a different response.

The conscious mind has a responsible job consisting of three tasks.

The first task is to observe and analyze the information that enters the brain through our senses seeing, hearing, feeling, smelling and tasting.

The second task is to observe and analyze the automatic reactions coming from the subconscious mind.

The third task is to observe and analyze the thoughts and beliefs already stored in the subconscious mind.

Because of these responsible tasks, the methods described below are meant to develop and train the prefrontal cortex home of the conscious mind.

The method consists of practicing a continuous routine of Focus - Action – Reflection combined with the Two-Step technique consisting of step one, prolonged pointed attention and step two, vivid creative imagination.

The Routine of Focus – Action – Reflection

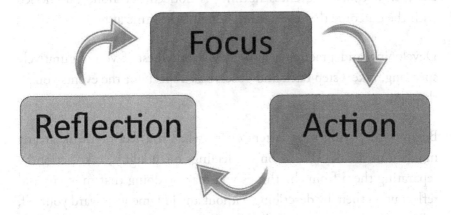

Focus-Action-Reflection

The purpose of this routine is to recognize and replace unsupportive thoughts, beliefs, habits and expectations and develop and instill a supportive and realistic self-image.

Awareness plays a key-role throughout this process.

Changing Life for the Better Begins with Awareness

The routine of focus, action and reflection begins with awareness, the state of *conscious* alertness that prevents thoughts, feelings, beliefs and expectations from passing unquestioned.

We have approximately 60,000 thoughts every day. About 95 percent of these thoughts recur on a daily basis and because the brain finds it easier to access negative memories, about 80 percent of these thoughts are negative. Just consider the sad impact these figures have on our daily living if we allow them to direct our actions and ultimately our life.

As mentioned before, awareness is the first condition necessary for change. Without awareness nothing is noticed, let alone questioned with the outcome that everything remains the same at best.

Developing and practicing awareness works best if you, figuratively speaking, take a step back and observe as a spectator the events you go through.

Begin with paying more attention to what you feel or think at any moment of the day. Focus on the feelings or thoughts, take action by separating them from the things you may be doing that moment and reflect upon them by describing without any judgments toward yourself, others or the environment what the feelings or thoughts are all about.

Reflect upon their true value and answer the question whether the thoughts or feelings are consistent with your intentions in life.

The process of reflecting begins with questions such as "why do I feel…, why do I think…, why do I believe I can't…, why do I believe I don't…, why do I always…?"

Translated to living a healthy life style of which eating healthy food and regular exercising are an indispensable part, the questions could sound like:

"Why does the thought of sweating and panting when exercising makes me feel uncomfortable while I know that sweating is the best way to remove toxins from my body and panting tells me that I am improving my stamina?"

"Why do I think I don't like lifting weights even though I understand that resistance training helps me to improve and/or maintain my strength?"

"Why do I eat food that I know harms my body and mind, and makes me feel guilty afterwards?"

"Why do I think a certain food is good/bad for me?"

"Why do I so often think negative about myself?"

"Why do I believe I can't lose weight?"

"Why do I believe I don't have time to exercise?"

"Why do I always compare myself to others?"

These are just a few examples. The list with questions could go on forever and expand to every aspect of your life.

The next step is asking yourself questions such as:

"And do I have a sane reason why I should think, feel, believe and act this way? How and where did I get these ideas? Could I be wrong? What would happen if I took a step back and seriously question the true value of these thoughts, feelings, expectations and beliefs? What would my conclusion be?"

In other words, answer the question whether you can identify thoughts, feelings, habits and expectations that don't support your intentions in life and need to be replaced.

Whatever you believe is possible in life forms the basis of all your choices. It is the sum of all your choices that formed your identity or self-image and comfort-zone and brought you to where you are now in life.

If you are not content with your self-image and where you are in life, it is good to realize two things. First, whether you believe it or not at this stage, you are holding beliefs and expectations in your mind that are holding you back from achieving your goals. Second, because you now understand how the mind works you have the ability to replace the unsupportive beliefs and expectations and change your life for the better.

It is our task to search our mind to find out which beliefs, values and habits are rationally sound and true, and we should never allow irrational beliefs, values and habits to pass unquestioned and get hold of us, not even for a while.

This is a task you'll always be performing since you'll experience new events every day and also need to continuously re-evaluate your current thoughts, beliefs and values and question whether they still help you achieving your goals.

Begin with writing down thoughts and feelings about topics mentioned above that may have resulted in beliefs, habits and expectations that no longer serve you and therefore need to be replaced. Next formulate your answers and comments.

The format of this exercise is as simple as this table below.

Question: "Why do I eat certain food that – although it makes me feel good – I know harms my body and mind, and gives me a bad feeling afterwards?"
Your Answer:

Using pen and paper or a computer helps to organize your thoughts, allows you to quickly read back what you have written and makes it easier to add or alter text whenever you want to. Nothing is set in stone. When you have made your first draft, put the notes away for a while and get back to them a few hours later or the next day. Coming back to what you have written with a different state of mind will give you new insights to further define your views.

In case you don't think it necessary to use pen and paper for this exercise, ask yourself why? Why do I think it is not necessary? Is it because I honestly believe that the results I get from this exercise will be the same regardless of whether I use pen and paper or just my mind? Or is it because that automatic response patterns in my head, influenced by my current beliefs, don't recognize using pen and paper as consistent with previous responses in similar circumstances and therefore reject it?

Succumbing to automatic responses means you're not really present and not engaging your conscious mind. This will result in doing things the same way you always did and will result in things remaining the same.

In other words, not using pen and paper dramatically diminishes the chances of developing a well-defined fresh view on certain believes and discovering new insights.

The exercise is inspiring and fun to do because you'll start a dialogue with yourself that opens doors to new places in your mind. You do the exercise at your own pace and feel safe because nobody will be looking over your shoulder and no one will ever see what you have written.

It would even be better to do the exercise on your own because if you discuss any of what you have written with others, chances are that their views and comments will influence you.

Of course, you won't be using pen and paper the rest of your life to contemplate your beliefs and habits. At one point the exercise has become second nature and therefore an automatic routine.

Do the exercise diligently. Shoddy work leads to shoddy results. Grab a sheet of paper whenever you run into more complex issues, jot down what comes to mind and come back to it later to add and adjust as much as you feel you need to. Nothing is ever set in stone.

Introducing the Two-Step Technique

What is the exact role of the Two-Step technique of step one, prolonged pointed attention and step two, vivid creative imagination in the process of replacing unwanted thoughts, feelings, beliefs and expectations?

To answer this question it is good to do summarize the main topics we covered so far.

The subconscious mind is impersonal. It takes in information, questions nothing and can't tell real from imagined.

The more emotionally charged experiences, the better memories and patterns of thinking, feeling, believing and expecting become ingrained.

The conscious mind living in the prefrontal cortex is only able to evaluate information if we consciously engage it.

Not consciously engaging our conscious mind means that information, good and bad, entering our brain via our senses has a free pass to our subconscious mind. It also means that automatic reactions, wise and unwise, coming from the subconscious mind have a free pass to the outside world.

It is through consciously engaging our conscious mind that we have the ability to reflect upon and replace ingrained negative automatic patterns of thoughts, beliefs, expectations and habits stored in the subconscious mind.

With these points as foundation it will be much easier to persist in applying the techniques that follow. The effort you will put in from now on will be well spent and consistently contribute to building a supportive self-image and replacing the beliefs and habits that till now have been in your way.

Like muscle tissue will grow in strength and size when it repeatedly works against a meaningful resistance, so will brain tissue form new patterns of thoughts, beliefs, habits and expectations when it is repeatedly stimulated.

No need to question these processes, if done correctly, the desired results will always follow.

Engaging our conscious mind with the goal to replace ingrained negative automatic patterns of thoughts, beliefs, expectations and habits stored in the subconscious mind requires applying a method that comprises prolonged pointed attention, and vivid creative imagination.

Let's begin with prolonged pointed attention.

Prolonged Pointed Attention

Prolonged implies repetition, repetition and repetition. Pointed attention means keeping yourself glued to the subject you're dealing with and the desired change you want to establish. Repetition creates and strengthens new neural pathways or brain patterns with supportive beliefs and weakens at the same time existing neural pathways with negative beliefs since they are no longer used.

The substance that plays a key role in this process is myelin, a whitish insulating sheath wrapped around the axons of many nerve fibers, forming an electrically insulating layer with the function to increase the speed at which impulses move. By repeatedly pointing your attention intensely on specific thoughts, feelings and beliefs you're activating that one specific pathway over and over again and stimulate the production of myelin.

This process is comparable to the process of forming new muscle tissue that occurs when muscles work repeatedly against a meaningful resistance.

This makes prolonged pointed attention so important. The benefit of understanding this automatic physiological process is that you don't have to question whether it works. The fact you know it works is very motivating because you can rest assured that every effort you will put in will inevitably bring you closer to your goals.

I understand that even though motivating, it is still easier said than done in this world where we feel ourselves pulled apart by the numerous tasks, responsibilities and obligations that ask for our attention.

But what does that mean? Does that mean that you therefore can't and therefore don't have to put in any effort to fix your attention to a specific subject? Of course not!

There are various ways to deal with this problem. The most commonly known technique most people think of when it comes to focusing attention and avoid distractions is meditating. This indeed is a very effective tool. All successful people, from athletes and artists to business people meditate because it makes them feel and perform better.

Most people don't meditate because they don't have the time, feel awkward when they do it, don't feel anything happen or feel that their mind is going all over the place with the most unexpected thoughts coming up that keep coming back no matter how often they try to re-focus.

I could say here that you can spare ten minutes per day, that you don't need to feel awkward when you are somewhere alone and that it is not mandatory or necessary to feel something. I could add that it is totally normal that if your mind is used to working at high speed most of the day, it will probably behave the same when you meditate.

Point is that you probably already know that but for some reason don't allow it to surface.

The first thing you do when objections come up is being aware of their presence. Then, instead of giving in, contemplate the true nature of your objections. In other words, question yourself whether you have a sound reason for giving in to your objections or that is to save yourself from discomfort.

Ask yourself "am I really right when I believe that meditation can and will never work for me because……………, fill in the blanks, although I know that if it works so well for so many other people, it can make a positive change in my life as well?"

What you want to accomplish with this question is figuring out whether your objections are the result of clear thinking of your conscious mind or that your subconscious mind is hijacking your conscious mind by making the latter fabricate excuses to justify the emotional reactions of the former.

The routine Focus – Action – Reflections is the method to deal with thoughts like these, and this process can go really quickly. Already asking the question may bring you straight to the conclusion "okay, I need to do this because I know that it will make me feel and perform better. What can I do to make it work for me?"

The answer begins with realizing that there is no one-method-fits-everybody solution. You are unique which means that the meditation technique you are going to develop needs to be unique. This sounds obvious but it is one of the reasons why most people fail at making daily meditation part of their life.

Most people are impatient and just want to get it going. They go online, choose a method they find most appealing, do it a few times, and then stop because that particular method didn't really fit with what they expected.

Another experience stored in the subconscious mind confirming the thought that they can't do what others can, leaving them behind disappointed and discouraged.

Therefore, instead of looking for a meditation practice you can just grab off the shelf develop your unique own practice.

Keep in mind that the goal of any form of meditation technique is to focus your attention on replacing unsupportive feelings and thoughts that lead to unwanted habits and expectations.

You might ask, "and how do you do that with a monkey mind, no time, no lust for feeling awkward or waiting for not knowing what and just wanting the benefits?"

The answer to this question is building your own unique meditation practice gradually.

Don't be disappointed. With gradually I refer to the form, not the result.

The form consists of two steps. The first step can be summarized with the words, if you can't beat them, join them. If you have racing thoughts that go all over the place, accept them for now and let them be. The only thing you will do differently from now on is being aware of your thoughts, notice those that are negative and replace them immediately for positive thoughts of any kind.

Positive thoughts create positive feelings that make you feel and look better, give you more energy, support an overall better performance and make you more pleasant to have around. The opposite is true too of course.

Feeling and looking good is the first step toward establishing a foundation for improving your self-image. Being aware of negative thoughts and replacing these for positive thoughts is a mental habit you need to install to open the doorways toward a relaxed and fulfilling life.

You can of course feel good and happy in many ways. Enthusiastic, energetic, grateful, excited, peaceful, lively, delighted, upbeat and joyful are examples.

Whenever during the day you think or feel negatively about yourself, about others, your past, present or future, you notice them, immediately put the brakes on and replace them for thoughts that match with the positive state you want to be in.

Think of a specific situation in the past when you felt good, happy, excited and so on. It doesn't matter if the context was entirely different, happened a long time ago, recently or today. Relive that moment as vividly as you can using all your senses while you stimulate and search for internal sensations.

To increase the effect of this technique, use a physical sign or movement to connect your feel-good state to.

The moment you're experiencing bliss or happiness as a result of reliving a good memory as vividly as possible, make a gesture, for example a circle with your thumb and index finger, and look intensely at that circle while you're fully aware of the positive mental state you're in.

The connection between that circle and your state of feeling good will serve as your safeguard when you need to recharge yourself with positive feelings in case negative feelings get a hold of you.

Summarizing this technique, follow these four steps:

- Decide in what sort of positive state you want to be.
- Think of a time you felt that way.
- Call up in your mind every detail of that memory and relive it as vividly as possible, using all your five senses.
- Create your personal safeguard by making a gesture such as making a circle of your thumb and index finger and put all your attention on that circle to connect it to the positive feeling.

Use this simple and popular technique every time negative thoughts show up in your mind and consider your good, happy, energetic, peaceful, joyful memories to be your safeguard.

Essential is to not just try to push the negative thought away, for that keeps your mind focused on negative thinking with the likely result that once you managed to remove one negative thought another negative thought instantly takes its place.

Therefore, focus on the negative thought or feeling and then immediately reach out for your safeguard and overwrite the negative thought with one that makes you happy, strong, confident, and so on. And if one happy thought becomes a bit stale over time, create a new one and another one. There are no rules when it comes to creating thoughts that make you feel good and support you in achieving your goals.

Apply this technique with gentle persistence. Replace from now on any negative thought or memory that comes up for a thought or memory that makes you feel good and then hold on to your safeguard. No planning or preparing, flip the switch, allow happy thoughts to come in and know that it will go easier every time. It eventually evolves into a habit that automatically comes into action whenever a negative thought appears.

Of course, I don't know where you are in life right now, what your life looks like, and I also don't know about your past experiences. And of course, it will be impossible to feel your best all the time. We all will meet with circumstances that have great emotional impact and put us through a period of grief. A reality of life nobody can escape. At one point however we all will have to bring up the strength, courage and responsibility to put ourselves together and embrace life again.

Having said that, you need to be careful that you don't keep overwriting negative feelings that are a result of experiences you have not yet fully dealt with and that keep lingering in your subconscious mind. That would get the character of fighting the symptom without addressing the underlying issue which would put you at risk for making yourself ill. If you know that you carry memories from experiences with you that you cannot resolve on your own, look for people or recourses that can help you.

From the moment you feel back on your feet again, it will depend on the decisions you make where you will be tomorrow, the day after and so on.

Negative thoughts or feelings won't serve you today and will never get you anywhere near your goals. Being upset with yourself won't help you and being upset with someone else will only hurt you, never the other. Also, being upset about a situation you probably can't even remember a few months from today doesn't make much sense either.

Let go, set yourself free and follow the recommendations below.

- Be kind, tolerant and forgiving to yourself and others
- Replace negative judgments about other people and their behavior for the best possible explanation you can think of
- Think positively about others and expect other people to think positively about you
- Genuinely be interested in others and what happens around you and let go of facts you cannot control
- Think, feel and act like the person you want to be
- Have in general an optimistic and positive view and be genuinely willing to see beauty in what surrounds you
- Count till ten. You don't have to respond to everything that comes to you
- Feel happy and smile often for the simple reason that you can't think of any other way to feel or to do

It may sound a bit bold but this is not the place to cut corners. Bring yourself back to this routine every time you become aware that you let it slip. Pick it up again while being kind and patient with yourself.

What may help is that you can even have fun with it. It sometimes can be really hilarious to observe and realize what you are thinking. There is a lot of value in the saying "don't take yourself too serious."

Talk to yourself with a positive attitude when you are on your own, for instance in your car. When you catch yourself with thoughts in your head that only produce feelings of frustration, anger, sadness and so on, ask yourself out loud if it wouldn't be much nicer and beneficial to come up with something positive?

Sure you can and sure you will. Will anybody or any situation get better if you submerge yourself in thoughts that make you feel miserable? If not, do yourself a favor, rely on your safeguard and think of something that makes you feel better. What also helps is to do things that make you feel better. Think of sitting straight up, taking a deep breath, singing and smiling. Combine all four for the best results and notice positive feelings and thoughts flow into your mind.

"Sometimes your joy is the source of your smile, and sometimes your smile is the source of your joy" – Thich Nhat Hanh.

Find something to remind you of this technique in case you are afraid that in the hassle of the day you may forget to apply it. Use a wrist band, a screen saver or whatever else works for you.

And consider this. Suppose you begin your day worrying whether you will be on time at the end of the day to pick up your child at the day care, catch your train or see that important game on TV. Do you need to remind yourself of that? Of course not! No matter how busy you are, you will never forget to bother about that important thing at the end of the day. Why not give this phenomenon a positive twist and apply it to the technique above?

In other words, it will almost be impossible to not become at least a few times during a day aware of negative thoughts or feelings. Realize that they don't serve any other goal than to make *you* miserable, and then decide that they must be replaced immediately, which is what *you* will do.

After a few days you'll notice that the negative thoughts or feelings become a reminder in themselves and that you catch yourself halfway the first negative thought. Put your safeguard in place and continue with words that radiate respect, joy and love toward yourself and your environment.

The four other things you will notice is that you will actually begin to feel better, behave more positively, that the speed of your mind begins to slow down and that it also becomes easier to focus your attention. Notice and recognize these effects and use them as a step up for more successes.

Once you feel that the routine of positive thinking becomes more ingrained, it is time for the next step.

Adding the Power of Vivid Creative Imagination

Combining prolonged pointed attention with the technique of vivid creative imagination forms the winning team through which you can work consistently toward creating a healthy self-image and life style you can maintain for life.

To maximize the power of vivid creative imagination it is important to choose a method that helps with further developing and training your conscious mind. You can do the technique described in step one any time and place of the day, but for this next step it is recommended that you minimize distractions as much as you can and better eliminate them entirely.

This doesn't mean that you let go of the technique in step one. Keep using this technique every day for the rest of your life. With some time it will become such an automatic and effortless habit that you won't even realize you're doing it, you simply don't know better. Good for you and the people you live and meet with.

Minimizing and preferably eliminating distractions in order to reap the full benefits of combining prolonged pointed attention and vivid creative imagination requires a time and place you can be on your own. Same as with studying or with anything else that askes for your full attention, nothing much can be expected if you can't concentrate on what you're doing.

The first objective of combining step one and two is creating a self-image that at least includes the qualities healthy, strong, confident, caring, giving and forgiving, and a clear sense of direction.

The second objective is to establish and maintain a continuous routine of focusing your attention on your thoughts, feelings, beliefs and expectations, followed by reflecting upon their true value and deciding which to replace.

Remember that creating a sound self-image is an essential condition before you can successfully replace beliefs and habits that until today weren't consistent with your intentions in life.

A time and place you can be on your own for a few minutes every day can take any form that works for you. Whether you call it meditation or something else is not important. The goal is to combine prolonged pointed attention with vivid creative imagination.

Think of a form you can fit these two techniques into. Sitting in a chair or lying on a bed is what most people do. What also works for many people is a walk in nature or doing some simple routine work, in- or out-doors, which for obvious safety reasons doesn't include driving a car or participating in traffic in any other way.

The reason combining prolonged pointed attention with vivid creative imagination works so well is best understood when you realize that the stronger you feel emotions during an event, real or imagined, the better and faster neurological pathways or brain patterns associated with the memory of the event become ingrained.

Here's where the neurotransmitters dopamine and endorphins or anandamide, known as the bliss compound, come into play. These neurotransmitters are important for many body functions but what they have in common is that they give the feeling of pleasure.

The difference between these neurotransmitters is that dopamine is released in anticipation of an event, whereas the other two are released during the actual experience of an event.

Translated to eating it means that dopamine is released when you look forward to having an ice-cream and that endorphins and anandamide are released when you actually consume the ice-cream. The stronger the emotion involved in the event the more neurotransmitters are released and the better you will remember the experience.

When you realize that your brain cannot distinguish real from imagined, understand the role and function of neurotransmitters and know that the release of the associated neurotransmitters happens automatically, then you can feel assured that this technique will help you with ingraining the desired result in your brain as quickly and effectively as possible.

Search your body during your meditation practice for physical reactions of excitement such as elevated heart beat and breathing and cultivate these reactions to make the experience as vivid and real as you can. It works like a two-way street. A positive, happy, excited attitude sparks positive emotions and positive emotions lead to happy feelings and a positive attitude.

To maximize the outcome of the meditation practice you need a place and time for your own where you feel safe and can't be disturbed.

Time now to find a form and type you can use to put prolonged pointed attention combined with vivid creative imagination into practice.

We went over the form. Choose what works for you and think of a time of the day. I suggest somewhere in the morning as it sets your mind for the rest of the day. If you prefer to sit, keep your back straight. Sit with dignity so to speak. Breathe normally from your belly in and out through your nose as it relaxes the mind.

Begin with a few exhales that last a second or two longer than your inhales. It really helps to slow down, relax and prepare for the practice. You'll read more about nose breathing later in this book. For now it is enough to just follow these simple suggestions. Close your eyes and let your hands rest in your lap or on your knees.

Remember, at this point the meditation practice is not yet meant to change unwanted habits. This will be our focus in Part Two and Three of this book where we go into healthy nutrition and safe and effective exercising. The goal of the meditation practice we focus on at this stage is improving and strengthening your self-image.

Work toward your ideal self-image in small steps. With this I mean that instead of pointing your attention right away on the perfect and ideal you, you define how you would feel and look like after making your first small step, and point your attention toward that picture.

For this, define a picture of yourself that will be relatively easy to achieve. Keep your focus at this stage on intensifying the practice, experiences and results of step one.

The reason for doing this is two-fold.

Pointing your attention on an ideal self-image that may need a long time to achieve is not realistic, and what is not realistic will be rejected by your subconscious mind because you don't truly believe it. Therefore, picture yourself how you will look and feel after completing your first small step. What is realistic, is easy to believe and makes mixing the picture with emotion almost effortless. Keep in mind that you need the emotions to induce the release of the feel-good neurotransmitters that help you with strengthening the brain pattern associated with your new self-image.

Making small steps offers the opportunity to define a newer image of yourself every time, which you can then use as a new goal to work toward. The outcome of using small steps will be that the repeated release of feel-good neurotransmitters will keep you motivated to continue working toward your perfect and ideal you.

Picture a big white screen in front of you and project yourself onto the screen as how you look and feel now. Let this picture then disappear to the right, representing the past, and move in from the left side of the screen, representing the present, a picture of you after completing the first step. Keep your attention on this picture or image.

Do this as vividly and as detailed as possible to promote the release of the feel-good neurotransmitters, your big allies that support you in the process. To enhance the experience, go into the screen and into yourself and look out of the eyes of the new you.

Use all your senses. Look very carefully at all the details of your new picture and your environment. Feel your new body when you look at your new picture, feel it when you perform daily activities such as driving your car, walking up and down the stairs, wearing the clothes you like to wear and hear the compliments you will receive from those who are important to you.

The technique of vivid creative imagination works best when using all the five senses, seeing, feeling, hearing, tasting and smelling. The first three are the easiest to work with as illustrated above. Although smelling and tasting are a bit more difficult to work with, they too have their place. We will use these in part two about healthy nutrition.

Using affirmations is another way to reach our brain in order to replace unsupportive beliefs and improve our self-image. The affirmation below consists of three parts. The function of the second and third part is to reinforce the previous part.

Reading and saying the affirmation aloud isn't very effective because it requires combining two different brain activities. Instead, take the effort to record the affirmation so that you can concentrate on the one activity of listening to your own voice. Also, listen to the affirmation three to four times in a row. Of course, when listening to the affirmation, be sure to mix it with true emotion to maximize the desired effect.

Here's an example of an affirmation.

"I feel confident, happy and safe because I love and accept myself as I am and see myself as the person I desire to be. Because I am allowing only good thoughts to enter my mind, I begin to notice how much more relaxed and confident I feel throughout the day. I know with certainty that my positive thoughts make me feel and look healthier and more energetic and that I therefore perform at my best every day. This is what I am and this is how I feel and act every moment of the day."

"Because I remember every moment of the day to think of happy memories, thoughts and plans only, I realize how much my confidence and self-esteem grow stronger every day. I feel confident, have more energy, look forward with positive excitement to every new day and actively look for ways to create new possibilities and experiences I can make part of my life. I am aware that the uplifting energy I experience empowers me and naturally brings my actions in alignment with my intention to maintain a lifestyle that supports a rewarding and fulfilling healthy and happy life."

"I feel great and am joyfully on my way toward creating my victory."

Helpful Thoughts...

Begin simple and short in the beginning, and build up from a few minutes to 5 to 10 minutes per day. More important than a specific duration is a duration that works for you, which of course can vary per day as well. What is of importance too is that you do it every day so that it becomes a habit.

You may forget a day when you begin with the routine, so be it. Do it the next day and you'll be fine. Tick off on a calendar every day you did your practice and get a nice looking series of ticks. That will help to stick to the routine for you don't want to see gaps in your series of ticks.

People often feel disappointed when they do not experience something magic during their meditation practice. Expectations like these have become an ingrained truth in their mind because of repeatedly seeing images or hearing information that linked meditation to monks, monasteries and Buddha-like enlightenment.

The world of meditation and related experiences is bigger than this. The magic you can expect are the vivid imaginations of the new self-images that appear on the big white screen you picture in your mind. These pictures combined with the emotions you will feel and cultivate are all the magic you need.

Combine prolonged pointed attention with vivid creative imagination and focus on what you imagine and how you feel without judging. Keep in mind that the practice is a tool, not a goal in itself and that there is no pressure.

You will experience the real benefits of the practice when you feel more relaxed and in better control the rest of the day. This is the real purpose of the practice. Therefore, see your practice as part of the day and not as a separate event. Allow feel-good neurotransmitters to flow and hold on to feeling good, relaxed and in control throughout the day.

At the end of each practice, take a few moments to reflect upon the practice to see if there are ways to improve the experience.

Work diligently and persistently and trust the process to work. It will work, so let it work. Give yourself the time you need and simply accept it when things sometimes don't go the way you had in mind.

Willpower is a word that often enters the picture when things need to get done. Willpower is fine but not used negatively in the form of attack or punishment. This strategy leads only to stress reactions with all the well-known consequences. Willpower is part of our conscious mind and when you realize that the subconscious mind is much stronger, you will understand that following the strategy of attack or punishment can only lead to failure.

Instead, master your willpower and use it in a positive way. First focus on the situation and accept it the way it is. Then take some time to reflect upon the situation so that, with a relaxed mind and body, you can take the wise decisions that will bring you further. Once you have taken the wise decisions you can guide your subconscious mind gently, patiently and persistently through the process of learning new supportive behavior.

Think of helping a toddler making its first steps. You patiently and gently encourage the child to try it again, and again. You never worry and simply trust the process because you know with certainty that one day the child will master the skill and make its first steps.

Learning new skills or replacing unsupportive beliefs, habits and expectations all have in common creating new neural pathways or brain patterns. It is in the nature of this mechanism that results don't come overnight.

It is a common saying that it takes on average 21 days to learn a new habit. Truth of the matter is that nobody is average and that the actual time needed for learning new habits depends on the nature of the habit and the effort put in.

Making the meditation practice a natural part of your life is not optional but a responsibility to honor and express your free will and to create a self-image that provides a solid foundation for building a rewarding and fulfilling life for yourself and the people you live and meet with.

Putting an End To: "Yes, But..." and Procrastinating

Understanding the processes in your brain and knowing how to master these processes makes fun of objections and excuses. No matter where you are in life, you now have the tools that help you staying in charge and giving your life the direction you desire.

Awareness is the first condition for change. Focus on where you are in the moment; what you are doing, thinking, saying and feeling, and then ask yourself if where you are is where you want to be physically, emotionally, mentally, spiritually.

Define every time what improvements you can make, implement the action-steps and reflect upon their effects on how you feel, think and behave. Keep repeating this routine to keep progressing.

Be aware of objections and excuses that come up in your mind and often begin with "yes but", as their only goal is to hold you back and to keep you where you are. Whatever comes after yes but often sounds like a knock down argument you have to succumb to, which is what most people do.

Objections and excuses begin as emotions coming from your subconscious mind. To avoid conflict, your conscious mind will search and find a justification for giving in to the emotions of the subconscious mind. This is the reason why excuses sometimes sound a bit silly.

From my experience I know that I can present a list with hundred reasons to do something, explain extensively about the benefits followed by seeing them all swept away with a 3-second response that begins with "yes but".

Yes but are words that from today on must let the bells ring in your head and make you stop to focus and reflect upon the true value of those words.

The most frequently uttered objection is "I don't have the time now, perhaps later". Believe me, you have the time, even if you have a busy job or business and live alone with three kids. Point is you need to find the time. A little exercise will help.

Grab a sheet of paper and write down in 15-minute segments what you do during the 7 days of a week. Review what you have written at the end of the week and see which activities you can delegate, re-organize, combine or terminate. This "Time-Bender" exercise is an exercise you can do on a regular basis to find out if and where you can do better, to sharpen the saw so to speak.

The format of the exercise looks like this.

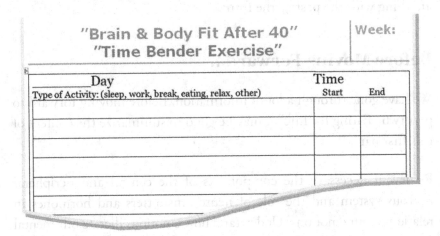

Time Bender Exercise

At the end of this book you'll find an example you can use to do this exercise.

Procrastination is another common pitfall. "I'll begin in the new year, after the vacation, a birthday" and so on is what these type of excuses sound like.

Waiting for the right time to put effort in making changes to establish healthy lifestyle habits is waiting for a time that will never come. It is never the right time, there is always something going on that will be in your way, if you allow it to be. You can't wait for the right time to arrive, you have to create it yourself.

Living a healthy lifestyle is a priority you cannot postpone until later. The clock keeps ticking and you can't allow feelings, thoughts, beliefs and habits to remain in place that make you feel unsatisfied and will only make things worse in the future.

Making the right decisions every day and throughout each day requires from us that we always be aware of where we are in the moment. Our conscious mind can only respond to the present moment. It cannot do anything with the past or the future.

Before Moving Forward...

We have gone through a lot of information. Before moving forward to part two "Eating for Life" it may be good to summarize the content of this first part.

Review if necessary the components of the central and peripheral nervous system and the role of neurotransmitters and hormones in relation to our emotions. Understand how emotions dictate our mental state and how they influence the metabolic processes in our body.

Review if needed also the role of the prefrontal cortex, home of the conscious mind, and the limbic brain, home of the subconscious mind, in the creation of memories, beliefs, expectations and habits.

The sum of all your memories, beliefs, habits and expectations, formed from your experiences, successes and failures ultimately determined how you perceive yourself, what your life looks like now and what it will look like in the future.

If you want to replace unsupportive habits, you need to look first for ways to change and improve your self-image since it is your self-image that forms the basis of your personality and determines the limits of your comfort-zone and what is possible.

Strengthening your self-image means working from the core and provides you with the confidence and sense of direction to correct the unsupportive habits.

You can change and strengthen your self-image by following the Two-Step technique.

Step One: prolonged pointed attention.

Recognize and immediately interrupt negative thoughts and feelings you have during the day and replace them for thoughts, feelings or memories that give you a supportive and uplifting energy.

Step Two: vivid creative imagination.

Vivid means that you mix the pictures you create in your mind with emotion. The stronger the emotion, the more effective the process of establishing new neural pathways will be. Make the event as real as possible by adding as many details as you can and using your senses hearing, feeling, seeing, smelling and tasting.

Small steps keep the images you create of yourself realistic, and therefore easier to believe. Small steps also keep the process fresh. Every time you feel excited about looking forward to completing a next step, dopamine will keep you motivated in anticipation of completing that step and endorphins and/or anandamide reward you with feeling good about yourself when you completed the next step.

The main purpose of the meditation practice is to set your mind for the day and to feel confident, centered and in control during the day. Repetition is king. Learning happens by trial and error and progress is per definition never a linear process. Going slow is never a problem. Keeping yourself in the process of learning and growing is all that matters.

You are unique and your own expert, so do not look for others you can compare yourself with, there simply aren't any.

Dare to make mistakes and expect setbacks. They are a natural part of the process and come with valuable information. There is no failure, only feedback. Make an inventory of possible events that might get in your way and think ahead of strategies to successfully deal with these setbacks.

Stick to the routine of Focus – Action - Reflection and begin every new meditation practice with a clean slate while cherishing the good experiences.

Focus, trust on the process and let go of the outcome. Stay away from questioning and judging yourself once you have set out your course as these negative thoughts can only initiate a stress-reaction.

A first condition for developing and training the mind to get the most out of the techniques outlined in Step One and Two is a continuous supply of healthy nutrients and oxygen and the removal of waste. This is the moment that the "Triangle of Good Health" enters the picture.

The Triangle of Good Health

The triangle of health consists of a strong, confident and secure mindset combined with healthy eating habits and effective exercise routines, each of them providing a foundation for the others.

A healthy and fit body facilitates optimal digestion, assimilation, brain health and brain function.

A healthy self-image creates a secure and supportive mindset and serves as a foundation for establishing healthy eating and exercise habits.

Healthy nutrition builds a healthy and fit body and brain, enabling both to function at their best.

The three components are of equal importance as illustrated with the image below.

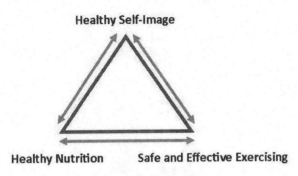

Triangle of Health

The common recommendation to move more and eat less in order to improve one's health and fitness assumes that the mind immediately understands and accepts healthy life style decisions and acts accordingly. It simply doesn't work that way.

Restating what I wrote at the beginning of this book; everything begins, ends and begins again in the head, brain and mind. Regardless of what you want to achieve in life, you need to begin with your mind.

If you have gone through the content of this first part and are consistently applying the techniques and suggestions in a manner that works for you, you have established a solid foundation to once and for all keep you on track toward achieving your goals.

The purpose of Part Two and Three is explaining the benefits for body and mind of healthy eating and safe and effective exercising and providing you with a sound plan for establishing eating and exercise habits that will consistently help you with achieving and maintaining your personal health and fitness goals.

I hope and trust you'll find it an exciting journey. The rewards of your efforts will be enormous. Not only will you look and feel so much better, you will have established a new lifestyle that allows you to perform at your best in every aspect of life.

Part Two

"Eating For Life"

"The food you eat can be either the safest and most powerful form of medicine or the slowest form of poison."

-Ann Wigmore

Health, the Foundation of Our Existence

Health is the first condition necessary to help us create the type of life we want. The first phase of our life is about growing, learning and preparing for adulthood. The better we navigate through this phase, the better we can convert the skills and knowledge gained into success during the second phase of our lives. It is obvious that good health is essential during both phases. Any time health is impaired there is a price to pay such as having to work harder than you would if you were in good health in order to achieve the same results.

The same goes for the third phase of your life, the older adult years. Entering this phase of your life in a less than optimal state lowers your quality of life and shortens your life span.

Health and success go hand in hand. What we perceive as success nowadays is very different from that of our ancestors who lived as hunters and gatherers. Success in those times meant daily survival and the production of offspring that had a better chance of survival than the previous generation. Good health was the best formula for success, the best guarantee that DNA passed on to future generations would make them even stronger than before. This is the law of survival of the fittest.

Life today is still about survival of the fittest. The fittest have the best chance to create and live the life they desire.

When can we consider ourselves to be healthy?

The World Health Organization (WHO) defines health as a complete state of physical, mental and social well-being, and not merely the absence of disease or infirmity.

Despite the WHO's definition, when people discuss health, they mostly refer to physical health only, which makes sense considering the fact that it is the most tangible and conspicuous aspect of health.

If physical health would be the only aspect that played a role in health, then health would be synonym to homeostasis, the condition where all body functions work optimally, and the demand for energy easily meets with the supply of available energy.

What follows from this limited definition of health is that we wouldn't have to look further than optimizing our eating and workout habits to maintain overall good health.

But to maintain good health we need to consciously focus at other aspects as well and reflect to what extend they play a role in our overall health and well-being, individually and in relation to one other.

Other aspects of health beside physical health are:

- Mental/Emotional health
- Social health/Relationships

- Spiritual health
- Professional health
- Financial health

All six components of health are equally important and together form the "Wellness Wheel", a reference to complete health and well-being.

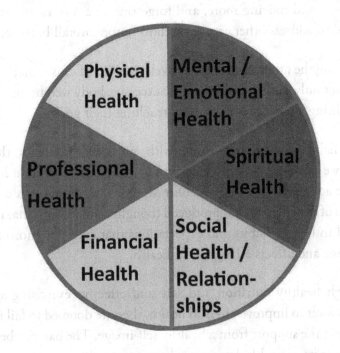

Wellness Wheel

A Delicate Balance

Since balance in our lives contributes to our overall feeling of well-being, all elements of health have to relate to each other in a way that serves us best.

Lack of balance within or between the six aspects of health eventually affects the entire wellness wheel and causes the weakest link to give out first. To illustrate this with an example, imbalance in mental health due to fear and anxiety is detrimental to our physical health, putting the body at risk for contracting something as simple as a cold or as serious as heart disease or cancer.

Being overweight is another example of a lack of balance. In our efforts to correct this state of imbalance, we often focus only on the physical aspect of the wellness wheel, resulting in the usual failing strategy of eating less and moving more, and forgetting to ask ourselves whether we need to address other areas as well to restore overall balance.

Neglecting the other aspects of the Wellness Wheel causes many people to fail not only in their efforts to lose excessive body weight, but also in maintaining a healthy weight upon reaching their goal.

Eating habits that are not in line with our body's needs are the first reason we become over- or underweight and are a result of a lifestyle we have adopted over the years. Our lifestyle is the result of a complex mixture of experiences that produced thoughts and feelings that in turn resulted in beliefs, habits and expectations that eventually formed our self-image and affects all aspects of health.

Although healthy nutrition and safe and effective exercising are the obvious tools to improve physical health, they are doomed to fail if both do not get the support from a healthy self-image. The balance between all six aspects of health determines how we perceive ourselves and how well we will be able to maintain and if necessary, regain physical health.

Bottom line: it is the balance between the six aspects of health that determines the quality of our self-image and therefore the quality of our life.

Healthy Nutrition, Safe and Effective Exercising and Our Conscious Mind

Recognizing what serves all aspects of your well-being is one thing, but actually bringing our actions and habits consistently in alignment with our intentions is something else. Despite our best intentions, distractions and excuses are always there to lead us astray and move us away from our intentions in life.

This is where our conscious mind part of our mental health, enters the picture. Without its support, nothing much can be expected from efforts to improve our overall health.

This underlines the importance of Part One, "Mastering Your Life", as the indispensable basis that creates the conditions for successfully generating and installing lasting lifestyle changes. In addition to its task to establish a sound and strong self-image, the role of the conscious mind in this part and in part three of this book is to support you with the next step; filling the gap between knowing and doing, the gap between intentions and results.

In other words, the second task of the conscious mind is to provide you with the tools, strengths and skills to cement habits into your lifestyle that supports, aside of your physical and mental health, also all other aspects of your personal wellness wheel.

But before we'll put the conscious mind at work to help replacing unsupportive lifestyle habits, we'll make an inventory of what healthy nutrition, the main subject of this part of the book "Eating for Life", is about.

The Five Circles of Healthy Nutrition

Nutrition is probably one of the most discussed topics by health and wellness professionals. Visit a bookstore or go online and search for information about healthy nutrition and you will feel yourself probably blown away by the available information.

Wouldn't it feel like heaven on earth, I sometimes wonder, if aside from the amount of information, we could at least reach agreement about what kind of nutritional habit is best for the body?

That indeed would be nice but that is probably not going to happen. Too many experts have an outspoken opinion about what is best to eat and what to avoid.

Similar to what I said about meditation practices, when it comes to healthy eating habits there is simply no one-advice-fits-all solution. Everybody is different which means that everybody's metabolic system is different. Eating habits that work for you may not work for someone else and vice versa.

More about this in detail later but the bottom line is that you have to be your own expert. Books, no matter how good, can only give you guidelines for healthy eating habits that at best cover 80 to 90 percent of the needs of your body.

Gender, age, body type, level of activity, mental state, environmental factors all play a role, which makes a one-advice-fits-all solution not a very workable approach. One may argue that good is good enough and that once 80 to 90 percent of a body's needs are covered everything will be fine, but the devil is in the details and that can play a significant role over time.

Instead of following external guidelines about what, when and how much to eat and drink throughout a day, you have to learn to interpret and follow the guidelines your body and mind give you, which they do, as you'll see. It is with the feedback you get from your body and mind you can easily make the course corrections to keep your intentions aligned with your goals.

It is my intention to bring with this book the whole discussion about nutrition back to the basics, back to simplicity. Healthy eating isn't that complicated nor should it be.

Therefore, instead of presenting you with my version of the 10 commandments with regard to healthy nutrition, you will read about healthy nutrition looked at from five perspectives; "Quality", "Quantity", "Timing", "Balance" and "Mastering eating habits".

Each of these five perspectives or circles of healthy nutrition begin with the fundamentals and build up to a point that you will automatically begin to connect the dots, meaning that you will see how things work and how they relate to one another.

Through this you'll make yourself part of the process, take charge and make the right choices that will help you with developing eating habits that bring you closer to your goals.

I recommend to first concentrate on the individual components "Quality", "Quantity", "Timing", "Balance" and "Mastering Eating Habits" outlined below and then on their connection.

Quality Quality forms the core of healthy nutrition. It refers to the quality of the food and fluid we consume. Everything we consume must be of optimal quality to support the functions of our bodily systems. Eating food of inferior quality is like building a house of inferior building materials and makes working on the other four components of healthy eating hardly worth the effort.

Quantity Eating healthy is important but too much or not enough never good. It is crucial that we feed our body with just the right amount of food and fluid for maximum performance.

Timing Timing answers the question when to eat and how to ensure that we have the right type of food available when we need it.

Balance Balance covers how to compose our meals to ensure that what we eat and drink is in line with the needs of our body. It is essential to realize that matching total energy intake with total energy output is only half the story.

Since the type and level of our activities typically vary throughout the day, it is important to match the *type* of food and fluid intake with the *type* of physical activity. For instance, when performing activities that are physically demanding, we need food that releases its energy quickly, whereas when we are not that active we can do with food that releases its energy at a slower rate.

Balance also refers to importance of eating and drinking in line with one's personal metabolic optimum. No metabolic system works exactly the same. Some work fast, others slow, some have a preference for certain nutrients whereas others may be intolerant to the same nutrients. Milk is a good example. Some people feel energized after drinking a glass of milk, whereas others may feel bloated and even nauseous. Understanding one's unique metabolic optimum and learning about the nutrients it thrives on, helps with staying energized and maintaining a healthy body weight.

Mastering Eating Habits Unless we manage to master the processes in our mind and teach it to respond with habits that support the body in its function, we keep spinning our wheels and remain trapped in a detrimental lifestyle. The aim is to bring balance to body and mind such that they support each another.

Balance among all six aspects of health is not something that can be achieved and maintained with the short term goals and actions often suggested by fad diets. Health stays with us a life time and that makes maintaining good health a long term endeavor.

Guess who enters the stage here? That's right; the conscious mind in the role of the chief conductor of the orchestra called our subconscious mind. In this fifth circle "Mastering Your Eating Habits" it is up to the conscious mind to compose a masterpiece from the four circles "Quality", "Quantity", "Timing" and "Balance" and to take the leading role when it is show time.

Translated to daily living it means that it will be the responsible task of your conscious mind to:

- Reflect upon the information in each of the four circles and decide what is relevant and consistent with your intentions in life
- Work out a strategy that consists of formulating new habits that are in alignment with your health and fitness goals
- Guide the subconscious mind through the process of implementing the new habits
- Be aware of the automatic reactions of the subconscious mind related to the new habits
- Apply the ongoing routine of Focus – Action – Reflection until the new habits have become ingrained

This may sound difficult but it is not. Exercises in this part of the book will help you to make an inventory of your current beliefs and habits with regard to eating and which of them need to be replaced.

After deciding which of those are not consistent with your goals and defining new ones that are, you will read how you can apply the same Two-Step technique of prolonged pointed attention and vivid creative imagination, used in Part One, to create a sound and solid self-image and to replace the habits you want to let go of.

This is a good moment to remind you to keep practicing the steps one, prolonged pointed attention using your safeguard, and two, vivid creative imagination, combined. Put a mark in your calendar every time you do the practice and see that you get a long series of uninterrupted marks. In case you miss a day say okay and begin again the next day.

Remember to make small steps, to think and behave as if you have already accomplished the steps and to trust and enjoy the process.

Making your happiness dependent on achieving a goal keeps you unhappy. The feeling of success after reaching a goal will only stay with you for a short time since there will always be a next goal to strive toward.

It is in the process that you spend most of the time of your life so you'd better enjoy it.

The First Circle of Healthy Nutrition, Quality

It is no surprise that low quality education for our kids, low quality gas in our cars, low quality building materials for our houses all lead to low quality results. Food is no exception. Eating low quality food leaves the body no other choice than to create energy and to build and maintain body tissue from inferior quality fuel and building blocks. The inevitable result of this can only be an under-performing body and mind every hour of the day.

The body constantly renews itself but it can take a while before old and damaged cells die off and are replaced by new cells. To give a few examples, skin cells have a life span of about 21 days, red blood cells 120 days and bone cells up to 25 years.

It is a fact that a body, built from poor quality building blocks will not be able to live up to its potential and is susceptible to diseases. Consistently eating good quality food is the foundation of good health and the first condition to get the best out of life. Choosing good quality food and fluid is not always easy but becomes less difficult once you know what to look for and where to find it.

Processed, Non-Processed, Organically Grown

What your body thrives on is food that fits with its metabolic system. This begins with choosing non-processed food, or whole food. Non-processed food is the type of food your body recognizes as being biological correct and congruent with its internal systems because it is wired that way.

A balanced meal of non-processed food provides the energy to keep all internal systems functioning and contains all the nutrients your body needs for energy and building, repairing and maintaining body tissues.

Respecting how your body is wired, and eating and drinking accordingly means looking at nutrition differently from what we were used to since the existence of convenience food, also known as fast food.

Processed, convenience or fast food, seen from the mind's bliss point perspective is quick, cheap, easy, tasty and good looking and fits with our senses. It automatically assumes that what is good for our mind, is good for our body, no questions asked, with all ensuing consequences.

The problem with this food is that it is often loaded with extra sugars, salt, unhealthy fats and chemicals that make poor quality food taste, smell and look better and give it a longer shelf life.

The amount of chemicals used in processed food today exceeds the two hundred. Conversations about whether or not food additives are safe or harmful go back and forth. To avoid adding more confusion to the discussion, I recommend staying away from food additives as much as you can.

The question is not whether these chemicals are toxic to the body or not. What they all have in common is that they are foreign to the body. The best you may hope from food additives is that they do not harm the body, although many of them probably do, one way or another.

Other chemicals you cannot expect many health benefits from are pesticides. Pesticides protect fruit and vegetables against invaders such as insects, weeds, rodents, fungi and bacteria but have a negative impact on the neurological function and brain health of humans.

Although it is possible to wash off some of the pesticides from fruit and vegetables by soaking them in a mixture of water and salt or vinegar, there are a number of toxic remedies that can't be washed off. An example is Glyphosate, a widely used broad-spectrum systemic herbicide used to kill weeds. The word systemic means that the toxin goes into the system or cells of the vegetable or fruit and therefore becomes part of the plant.

Glyphosate is the active ingredient in Roundup and in 2015 classified by the International Agency for Research on Cancer (IARC), an arm of the World Health Organisation (WHO), as "probably carcinogenic to humans".

Genetically Modified Organisms (GMO), also known as Genetically Engineered (GE) or Genetically Modified (GM) food form a special category when it comes to food handling.

In an attempt to reduce the need for pesticides, techniques have been developed to modify the genetic blueprint of fruit and vegetables to make them more resistant to insects, fungi, other unwanted visitors and even pesticides. Reality learns that the use of pesticides hasn't declined but has increased considerably the past decade.

Apart from the toxins used, there is increasing concern about the long-term risks to human health of consuming GMO's. Scientists repeatedly warn that GMO food can create unpredictable, hard to detect side effects, including allergies, toxins, new diseases and nutritional problems. The most prominent GMO food are corn, soy, sugar, papayas, canola oil, zucchini and yellow squash.

You can recognize GMO fruit by checking the numbers on the little stickers on fruit or vegetables. If the number starts with an 8, you know that the fruit or vegetable is genetically modified. A GMO banana for instance carries the number 84011. On the other hand, if the number begins with a 9 then you know that the produce was grown organically. An organic banana will for instance carry the number 94011.

Any produce that has a sticker on it starting with a 4 tells you that it has been produced conventionally, meaning that it probably has been sprayed with pesticides.

Toxins and chemicals that affect your health are everywhere and certainly not in food alone. Think of cosmetics, shampoos and deodorants. Chemicals in these products are absorbed through the skin and can interfere with the body systems.

Flame-retardants are other known risks. They are present in clothing, furniture, carpets, car seats, baby products and in numerous other consumer goods.

It is hard, if not impossible to avoid toxins. The only way to deal with these threats is by avoiding them as much as you can through buying products that are as close to their original state as possible, starting with food.

The Bliss Point and the Brain's Reward Centre

As mentioned before, in their quest to realize the highest possible revenue, big food companies focus on what they refer to as the bliss point. This is simply the point at which we experience the greatest amount of craving stimulus due to the product's taste, smell and look. The more we crave a product, the more we buy and consequently the higher the company's profit margin. It is that simple. Don't look for moral issues.

The purpose of the bliss point is to trigger the area of your brain known as the reward centre, the same centre triggered after consuming alcohol, nicotine and narcotics. The result is that you feel good and desire more of the particular product. Sugar has the same effect on the brain, which is why it is so widely used by the food industry.

What triggers the reward centre of your brain and makes you feel good is not necessarily good for the rest of your body and can easily lead to imbalances in one's physical and mental health.

We can witness the common outcome of this picture every day around us. People can't resist fast food for reasons of convenience and comfort and react the next day with bursts of willpower to deal with the feelings of guilt and unwanted physical effects.

The result is a never-ending struggle between mind and body. Unfortunately, the brainstem, the part of the brain that harbours the reward centre also harbours our basic survival system and is therefore unbeatable in terms of strength and endurance. Thus, relying on willpower alone is playing a losing game.

Although most people understand the importance of changing their situation, very few are able to summon the strength and perseverance to actually implement the necessary changes and cement them into their lifestyle.

Food companies spend vast sums of money on research and marketing to connect consumers to food that is convenient, inexpensive and feel good. They have developed a wide range of formulas to reinforce the public's bliss points and keep them craving more.

Picture yourself as a consumer in a grocery store with a head full of obligations, responsibilities and a chronic lack of time. You can't see them, but opposite you, behind every product on a shelf, there is a legion of food scientists and marketers. The task of these people is to eliminate any form of resistance in you and to assure you that the best thing you can do for yourself and your family is buying their products.

Reading and Understanding Labels and Ingredients

Think from the manufacturer's perspective when you read the fancy words and see the funny images on packages on the shelves. Feel good emotions play a key role in marketing.

Don't buy a product based solely on what is on the front of the packages but check out the label and, especially, the ingredients too. Be careful, although food manufacturers are legally required to be honest about the ingredients in their products, they can be very creative in their choice of words.

Be wary of the following words on a package.

"Made with real fruit". This claim says nothing about the amount of real fruit in the product.

"95% fat-free". This means that the product contains 5% fat. The next question is what type of fat? You would be best to put the package back on the shelf if the label says trans-fats, partially hydrogenated fats, vegetable shortening or margarine.

"Zero trans-fats". This doesn't guarantee that there are no trans-fats in the product. Food manufacturers are required to list an ingredient on the label only if a product contains more than 0.5 grams per serving of that nutrient. This may not sound like much but it can add up quickly when you eat more products that contain trans-fats. More about trans-fats later in this chapter.

"Fat free". This statement on products that are fat free by nature like dates and 100% orange juice probably serves to distract your attention from ingredients that are less healthy.

"All natural ingredients". This claim tells you nothing. For instance, salt and sugar are both natural ingredients but they don't necessarily turn food into healthy products.

Healthy eating begins with staying away from food and fluid that are responsible for creating unwanted physical and mental effects. For thousands of generations non-processed food has provided us with all the nutrients our body needs to function optimally. It is only in the past few generations that we have begun to eat and drink food and fluid that have lead us to epidemic levels of life threatening chronic diseases such as cancer, diabetes, heart disease and obesity.

While understanding the importance of eating non-processed food is critical, actually making the switch away from eating mainly processed food is not so easy and requires an entirely different mindset. It is the purpose of this book will help you with that switch.

Where to Find Non-Processed Food?

You can find non-processed food mainly in the outer aisles of your supermarket. Main characteristic of non-processed food is that it usually contains just one ingredient.

Think of vegetables, fruit, meat, fish, dairy, nuts and seeds. Although they are in the outer aisles where you will spend most of your time when shopping, you will need to visit the inner aisles too for products like coffee, tea, spices and olive oil.

You need to be extra careful with your choices in the processed food sections. It is more important here than anywhere else in the supermarket to read the labels on the packages. The trouble with many of these labels is that they are often so small that you may need a magnifier to read them. Therefore this tip, keep a magnifier in your shopping bag.

Again, do not only check the food labels but also read the section on the packages listing the ingredients. Know that food producers only have to list ingredients on the labels if the product contains 0.5 grams or more per serving of that specific ingredient. There are plenty of ingredients you don't want in your system, no matter how minor or insignificant. A rule of thumb is to put a product back on the shelf when you read an ingredient that you can't pronounce, let alone understand.

To minimize the chance you'll consume ingredients that may be detrimental to your health is to eat only organically grown, non-processed food.

How Foreign Invaders Affect Your Health

Two quotes that will set the tone,

"all disease begins in the gut", and "death begins in the colon".

The first quote is from the Greek physician Hippocrates and the second from the Russian biologist and Nobel prize winner Elie Mechnikov.

Due to the work of science we know that up to 90 percent of all known human illness can be traced back to an unhealthy gut. The same is true for health and vitality.

The microbial organisms that reside in and on our body comprise bacteria, fungi and viruses and outnumber our body cells by a factor ten. We're looking here at about 100 trillion of those creatures, of which bacteria form the majority.

Imagine, these creatures lived already for millions of years on this planet before we arrived.

Put them all together and you could fill a half-gallon container.

About 10,000 species of microbes have been identified, but some experts argue that we have to give a name to another 25,000.

Think of this, each microbe contains its own DNA. For every human gene there are at least 360 microbial ones and most of them live in the digestive tract. We interact with these organisms and with their genetic material.

What makes humans so different from one other is *not* their DNA, for that is, apart from the few genes that determine characteristics such as hair color and skin, almost the same for everybody. No, what makes humans so different from one other is their microbiome, the total of microbiome flora that occupies the gut and interacts with our DNA.

Because the state of the microbiome is as vital to health as heart, lungs, liver and brain, you should look at it as an organ in and of itself.

Our microbiome plays a key role in our health. Some examples are:

-   assisting with the digestion and absorption of nutrients
-   forming a barrier against invaders such as bad bacteria, harmful viruses and parasites
-   working as a detoxification device; a second liver so to speak
-   making your gut the biggest immune system organ. This makes sense if you consider that, same as skin, the intestinal lining forms the connection with the outside world,
-   production of important enzymes, brain chemicals, vitamins and the feel-good neurotransmitter serotonin,
-   assisting in getting a good night's sleep,
-   through assisting in mastering the body's inflammatory responses reducing the chance for developing nearly all types of chronic diseases.

As mentioned, bacteria form the majority of our gut flora. Not all bacteria are good or bad, a healthy ratio would be 85 percent good and 15 percent bad. This healthy ratio is very important because all the bacteria together form an inner ecosystem that influences numerous aspects of health.

The bacteria in your gut communicate with one another and know when they outnumber other types of bacteria. This helps them to coordinate their defense and attack systems.

The gut also harbors the hundreds of millions of nerve cells forming the intestinal nervous system, or enteric nervous system, created from the same tissue as the central nervous system.

During fetal development, one part develops into the central nervous system while the other part "wanders off" and develops into the enteric nervous system. Containing 500 million neurons, which is more than in the entire spinal cord, the gut literally functions as a second brain.

Head and gut brain remain connected via a cable called the vagus nerve which runs from the brainstem to the abdomen. Vagus in Latin means wandering.

Information constantly goes back and forth between head and gut brain which means that they influence each other. Think of the butterflies you feel in your stomach when you are in love or the stomach ache you feel when you truly dislike somebody.

When the microbes in the gut stimulate the millions of nerve cells of enteric nervous system, the central nervous system becomes immediately informed.

No other body system is more sensitive to changes in the gut flora than the central nervous system, especially the brain.

The examples listed above illustrate what can happen when the gut flora becomes disrupted due to toxins, harmful bacteria and unhealthy food choices.

In short, a disrupted gut flora can make the brain sick and at the same time allow harmful invaders get passed their defense system and enter the blood stream.

From there virtually anything can happen ranging from brain diseases such as Parkinson's, multiple sclerosis, depression and dementia to heart diseases, autoimmune disorders and cancer.

Bottom line, your gut flora influences to a large degree your physical as well as your psychological health, which makes optimizing your intestinal flora a priority.

You can do a lot to keep your microbiome healthy by choosing for food your gut flora recognizes as biologically correct which is organically grown whole food, food raised without the use of antibiotics and hormones and good fats such as extra-virgin olive oil, nuts, seeds, avocados, coconut oil and butter.

Other ways to protect your gut flora are avoiding medication containing antibiotics as much as possible since they not only kill bad bacteria but also the good ones. Avoiding drinking chlorinated water also helps to protect your gut flora.

Helpful for improving and maintaining a healthy balance of the gut flora is eating fermented food such as sauerkraut, kefir, tempeh and pickles and probiotic yoghurts without added sugar or fruit.

A special place with regards to making healthy food choices deserves the discussion around grains, in particular wheat.

Bread is for many of us the food we have been raised with since it contains so many healthy nutrients. The point is that bread nowadays hardly resembles the bread our grandparents used to eat.

Hybridization methods have transformed grain over the past 50 years dramatically. This process has allowed producers to realize large-scale production, increase yield per acre, decrease production costs, decrease vulnerability to diseases and achieve greater resistance to drought. Grain may look the same on the outside as it did 50 years ago but there are mounting indications that the nutritional content of grain has changed dramatically, and not for the better.

Grains in general and wheat in particular are increasingly linked to excessive weight gain and numerous health problems.

The concerns related to wheat are two-fold.

75 percent of the complex carbohydrate in wheat converts into blood sugar more efficiently than nearly all other carbohydrate rich food, simple or complex. This effect can contribute over longer periods to weight gain.

About 10 to 15 percent of wheat is protein and 80 percent of that protein is gluten. Glutens are essential for the wheat plant to form new wheat plants and make wheat dough stretchable, roll-able and spreadable.

The concern with glutens is that they can damage the health of the small intestine and create a pathway for bacteria, harmful viruses, parasites and chemicals to enter the blood stream, with all the ensuing consequences outlined above.

Another concern is that just before harvest a great part of conventional grown wheat is sprayed with the herbicide Roundup, with Glyphosate as the active ingredient, to increase yield and make harvesting easier.

Achieving and maintaining good health means choosing quality food that create the right circumstances for your microbiome to do its job properly. Creating the right circumstances means only eating what the body recognizes and knows how to digest and process.

Keep in mind though that healthy nutrition alone can't do the job and that regular physical activity is essential to keep all body systems healthy and functioning at their best. We will cover this in Part Three.

More About Organically Grown

A step up from eating non-processed food is eating food that is organically grown and locally produced.

Organically grown food is produced with respect for product, the people that work with the food and the environment. Often it has a better taste and is produced without the use of pesticides, growth hormones and antibiotics. The best organic food is locally grown.

A common objection to organic food is that it is more expensive than food that is not organically grown. This may be true but there are ways to work around this. First, be sure that you buy products that are in season. Fresh strawberries are expensive around Christmas. Buying them in the summer and storing them in the freezer until Christmas is a good way to save money and it works for other food as well.

Another way to save money is to stay on the outlook for promotions. This is the perfect moment to buy extra and keep them in the freezer until you are ready to eat them. Purchasing organic food in season and in bulk can be more affordable than you ever thought.

The big pay-off for buying organically grown products is that you invest in your health, short term as well as long term. Investing in non-processed and preferably organically grown food can save you from developing minor and major health issues that inevitably lead to a loss of productivity, due to an under-performing body, wasting time seeing your doctor, spending money on medications and overall loss of quality of life.

Nutrients and Calories

All your body cares about when you eat are the nutrients that are in the food and fluid you consume. No matter how intricate the recipes or special the dishes, the only thing your digestive system can and will do is process whatever is consumed, utilize nutrients and dispose of the rest.

Nutrients are chemical components of food that are essential for energy, growth, cellular repair and regulation of metabolic functions.

Nutrients are divided in macronutrients and micronutrients.

The macronutrients are:

- carbohydrates, containing 4 calories per gram
- protein, containing 4 calories per gram
- fats, containing 9 calories per gram

The micronutrients are vitamins, minerals and water and don't contain calories.

Water is often also called a macronutrient since the daily requirement of this nutrient is so high compared to that of other nutrients.

Although the body creates energy from all three of nutrients that contain calories, the way your body creates energy is different for each of them.

The number one mistake people make when it comes to losing weight is thinking of nutrients only as sources of calories and concluding that you simply need to burn off more calories than you consume.

However, if you understand how the body treats the nutrients we ingest then the limitations of "calorie in, calorie out" become obvious. It is one of the topics we'll discuss in the coming chapter.

Carbohydrates

Carbohydrates are everywhere it seems. Some examples are sugar, bread, cereal, potatoes, spaghetti, all flour-containing items, juices, honey, beans, dairy products, canned soups, ketchup, sweet condiments and relishes.

Carbohydrates are the most easily accessible source of energy and therefore the ideal source of energy for muscle and brain function.

Carbohydrates and the Function of the Hormone Insulin

Simple carbohydrates have one or two units of sugar and are separated in two groups.

Monosaccharides are made of one simple sugar molecule. Most common examples are glucose, dextrose, fructose found in fruit, and galactose present in milk, whey and the human body for breastfeeding. Glucose and dextrose are biochemically the same. The difference is that glucose is the name for sugar in blood, and dextrose is the name for glucose produced from corn.

Disaccharides are made of two simple sugar molecules. Examples are sucrose or table sugar, composed of one molecule glucose and one molecule fructose, and lactose or milk sugar, composed of glucose and galactose.

Complex carbohydrates combine more than two units of sugar and are also separated in two groups.

Oligosaccharides form the first group. Examples are raffinose, a trisaccharide found in sweet potatoes, beans and beets, consisting of glucose, fructose and galactose. Oligosaccharides are also the result of breaking down polysaccharides.

Polysaccharides form the second group and can consist of more than 10,000 monosaccharides. They include starch, consisting of amylose and amylopectin as in bread, glycogen, complex chains of glucose stored in muscles and liver, and fiber or cellulose, the structural material in plants.

Simple or complex, all carbohydrates consumed eventually end up as a monosaccharide in the blood stream. The big difference between the two types of carbohydrates is the digestion time. Digesting simple carbohydrates is simpler and faster than digesting complex carbohydrates.

Although sugars contain the same amounts of calories, they are metabolized differently.

When the monosaccharide glucose enters the blood stream, the pancreas gland responds with the production and secretion of the hormone insulin. This hormone is an essential component of the metabolic system and functions as a key on the surface of body cells to let glucose enter.

Without insulin, cells are unable to pull in glucose to either store or use it as energy for various body functions. People with diabetes don't produce enough insulin and may need to inject insulin several times a day.

The other name for insulin is the storage hormone because it removes excess, and therefore toxic, levels of glucose from the blood stream.

Glucose entering the blood stream can go in two directions.

The first direction is to muscle and brain cells and other cells that either utilize the glucose right away for the production of energy or store it as glycogen, chains of two or more glucose molecules, for later use. The muscle cells in the average body can store about 200 to 400 grams of glucose in the form of glycogen while the liver stores about 80 to 120 grams. The former is for muscle function only, the latter to maintain normal blood sugar levels.

The second direction is to fat cells. This happens when muscle and other cells don't need glucose and have reached their storage limits. Insulin will then signal the liver and the fat cells to pull in the glucose from the blood stream. The fat cells metabolize the glucose and bundle the by-product of this process, glycerol, together with the fatty acids into triglycerides to store it as fat. The liver converts part of the glucose into glycogen and part of it as fat, and stores both.

The result of this glucose-insulin-fat deposition is especially visible in the abdomen. The bigger the belly, the poorer the response to insulin, since the deep visceral fat of the belly is associated with poor responsiveness, or resistance to insulin.

To cope with this situation the pancreas secretes more insulin, which in turn leads to more fat storage. Belly fat is a unique metabolic factory. It produces and releases inflammatory chemicals into the blood stream, cultivating diabetes, hypertension, heart disease, dementia, rheumatoid arthritis and colon cancer. Waist circumference is proving to be a powerful predictor of these conditions as well as of mortality.

Every time you eat carbohydrates, insulin is doing the same job. This is an endless process since insulin signals your body to create new fat cells every time they have reached their storage capacity.

Unless your body immediately uses up the glucose you take in as carbohydrates, it converts most of it into fatty acids and then stores it as body fat. This makes it important to balance your carbohydrate consumption with the type and level of your physical activity. You can read more about this topic in the chapter about the fourth circle of healthy nutrition, balance.

The treatment of the monosaccharide fructose is entirely different. Fructose doesn't influence your blood sugar and insulin levels but is metabolized by the liver that directly converts the fructose into fatty acids.

It is good to realize the evolutionary purpose of fructose, naturally occurring in fruit. The time of year for animals, and humans back in the days, to fatten up in order to make it through the winter is during end of summer and fall.

Fructose helps with the process of fattening up for winter in three ways.

First, it goes straight to the liver where it is converted into fatty acids, second, it blocks the release of the hormone leptin that normally sends out a signal to the brain that the body has eaten enough food and that it is time to stop, and third, it reduces activity levels.

Toward the end of summer and during the fall, animals eat as much as they can and reduce activity with the purpose to preserve energy and to build up a good layer of fat they can rely on during the winter months when not much food is available.

Meanwhile, the glucose that came with the fructose, raised blood sugar and insulin levels, pushed the body in a fat storing mode, and amplified the process of storing calories from other consumed nutrients.

It requires the release of specific enzymes to reverse this process of fat storage. These enzymes however, will only be released when both glucose and insulin levels are low, allowing the body to shift from fat storing into fat burning.

Fructose is present in almost all processed food, most often in the form of high fructose corn syrup (HFCS), a sweetener made from corn starch, consisting of 45 percent glucose and 55 percent fructose. As an example, a 12-ounce can of soda contains about 40 grams of sugar of which at least 20 grams is fructose.

Fructose is also present in fruit, but the amounts are relatively low. You will have no problem with staying below the maximum recommended intake of 25 grams per day if you limit yourself to eating 2 to 3 pieces of fruit. Nowadays, adults consume daily on average over 50 grams of fructose and adolescents over 70 grams.

The Myth Calorie-In, Calorie-Out.

Let's have a look at the official definition of calorie.

1 calorie, or 4.1868 joules, equals the energy that is needed to raise the temperature of one gram of water through 1 degree celcius.

And here is what the first law of thermodynamics states,

Energy can neither be created nor destroyed. It can only change forms. In any process, the total energy of the universe remains the same. For a thermodynamic cycle the net heat supplied to the system equals the net work done by the system.

This, at first sight, eliminates all discussion. A calorie is a calorie, no questions possible.

Translated to our daily eating and drinking, when we see on a package that 100 grams of a nutrient contains, for instance, 200 calories we are quick to conclude that if we don't burn all of those 200 calories the body will store any surplus as body fat.

Which eventually will be the fact, but before coming to that conclusion it is important to understand that the body doesn't treat all incoming calories equally.

The difference between the two simple sugars fructose and glucose offers a good example. Both are present in table sugar on a fifty-fifty basis and both contain per gram the same amount of calories.

Glucose will be used for muscle and brain function. If you don't take in too much of this substance and are fairly, most or all of it will be used up.

Fructose on the other hand goes straight to the liver where it is converted into fatty acids and shipped off to storage. As long as there is enough glucose present, your body will give priority to using the glucose and wait with calling the fatty acids coming from fructose into action.

This happens for two reasons. First because it is much easier to convert glucose into energy than fatty acids, and second, high glucose levels are toxic to the body, which means that your body gives priority to using up the glucose first.

The hormone insulin therefore signals the cells in your body to use up the glucose present in the blood stream first and prohibits the use of other sources of fuel, such as the fatty acids from fructose, by preventing the release of enzymes that normally promote the conversion of those sources of fuel into energy.

In other words, to prevent weight gain, limiting the intake of fructose is a good choice.

But the only way to realize that is by reducing your overall sugar intake since fructose almost always comes with glucose.

The bigger picture shows that although glucose and fructose contain per gram the same amount of calories, the calories in fructose are of bigger concern than those in glucose when it comes to weight gain.

Another example is the thermic effect of food (TEF), which stands for the amount of energy that is needed to process the food we consume.

On average, about 10 percent of the calories we take in are used for this process.

But there is a significant difference when looking at the three macro-nutrients carbohydrates, protein and fat.

Roughly 15 percent of the calories coming from carbohydrates are used to process this nutrient. The percentage for protein is between 20 and 30 and for fat between 5 percent. The actual percentage depends on factors such as type of food and the efficiency of one's metabolic system.

Of course, a calorie remains a calorie. The point again is that looking at calories from the perspective of to gain weight or not to gain weight, there is more to consider than the number of calories mentioned on the label on the package that contains the food.

The Dangers of Sugar

Limiting your intake of sugar is important not only to avoid weight gain but because sugar sets off reactions in your body that can be extremely harmful.

Sugar triggers the same reward center in your brainstem as does alcohol, narcotics and nicotine. Sugar is physically addictive. The difference between sugar addiction and narcotic addiction is mainly one of degree.

What tells you that you are addicted to something like sugar? Addiction comes in many degrees but becomes an issue when you can't control the desire for more after taking small amount, and when you notice withdrawal symptoms such as strong cravings, mood swings, irritability and headaches when you stop abruptly eating sugar.

Sugar in itself is devoid of vitamins, minerals or fiber. It is rapidly converted into fat or triglycerides and causes a tendency to overeat.

When you consume food that contains sugar, part of the sugar molecules lose their coherence and stick to all kinds of protein structures in the body. Examples are blood cells, lipoproteins, responsible for the transport of cholesterol through the body, collagen, the connective structure that keeps tissues together and beta cells, the cells in the pancreas that produce the hormone insulin and DNA.

Organs slowly disintegrate due to an excessive intake of sugar. This process, called the glycation process, ends when the intake of sugar ends but becomes irreversible when sugar keeps entering the body. The protein-glucose structures eventually turn into advanced glycation end-products (AGEs) and can set off serious health problems throughout the body.

Some examples:

AGEs stick to artery walls, cause permanent inflammation, compromise the function of the immune system and damage the protein in collagen and elastin, necessary to keep your skin elastic and firm. AGE's also prevent that insulin and cholesterol are utilized for body functions as a result of which they begin to stack up. Eventually, the artery system as a whole becomes affected and it becomes only a matter of time for cardiovascular diseases to appear.

Other harmful effects of AGEs are:

AGEs stick to white blood cells, preventing them to do their job, killing harmful bacteria. Only a few tea spoons of sugar in your tea or coffee is enough to reduce the function of your immune system with about 25 percent and a cake and ice cream for dessert may shut down the white blood cell activity for up to 5 hours.

A body that can't rely on a proper functioning immune system when it comes to fighting a simple cold or even a life threatening disease such as cancer, is playing a losing game.

Excessive sugar intake promotes the forming of wrinkles due to a loss of skin tissue elasticity and function, premature aging, weakening of eyesight, development of autoimmune diseases such as arthritis, asthma and multiple sclerosis, impairment of the DNA structure, osteoporosis, a decrease in insulin sensitivity, eventually leading to diabetes.

Since the entire human body is made up of protein structures, there is no organ or body function that can't get impaired from a continuous intake of sugar.

The list of consequences of excessive sugar intake is therefore almost endless. Other effects of excessive sugar intake are an increase in total cholesterol, triglycerides and bad cholesterol levels and a decrease in good cholesterol. Sugar has been connected to the development of many forms of cancer and mental diseases and conditions such as Alzheimer's disease and worsening of symptoms of attention deficit hyperactivity disorder (ADHD).

Sugar from carbohydrates, simple or complex, is an important source of energy for the body and contributes to optimal function of all body systems as long as the intake of sugar is in balance with the type and level of physical activity.

Sugar in itself isn't a bad nutrient. Problems arise when the intake of sugar is more than the body needs or can handle which is often the case in our modern society where the availability and consumption of sugary food is high and the level of physical activity is low.

Artificial Sweeteners Are No Alternative

Artificial sweeteners are much sweeter than table sugar. This creates the risk that your taste buds eventually become dulled and less receptive to natural sources of sweetness as in fruit, causing you to seek out sweeter and sweeter food.

Artificial sweeteners confuse your gut. The sweet taste sends out the signal that something high calorie is on its way but when that doesn't arrive, your gut utilizes the food inefficiently resulting in a number of effects that interfere with the body's hunger regulating systems.

One of these effects is the release of the hormone insulin. Calories or not, your body releases insulin as if you'd eaten sugar, setting off a desire to eat. In addition, since artificially sweetened food isn't as satisfying as real food because of its structure, you probably eat too much with all ensuing health consequences.

Lastly, artificial sweeteners can be made from corn, soy or sugar beets which are crops that have often been genetically modified.

The alternative here is table sugar or a natural sweetener such as Stevia. Even better, avoid added sugars in any form.

Your Focus: Complex Carbohydrates

As mentioned earlier, carbohydrates are everywhere. Almost all food contains carbohydrates, which makes it very challenging to eat the right amount and right type of carbohydrates.

A good start would be to avoid eating simple carbohydrates found in table sugar, candies, honey and all flour-containing items like cakes, bread and pastas for the reason that it requires hardly any time and effort for the body to convert these simple carbs into glucose and then into fatty acids. Once at this stage, the fatty acids only need to be bundled in three to end up as triglycerides and stored in the fat cells.

Your body stays in a storing mode as long as the insulin level remains elevated. Once your insulin level drops back to normal, the body shifts from storing mode to burning mode to use up what has been stored before. The burning mode in turn ends the moment insulin levels rise in response to a new load of simple carbohydrates.

When eating carbohydrates, it is generally better to focus on the complex carbohydrates as in vegetables, legumes and fruit. Vegetables in particular are dense and high in fiber, which causes a slow release of the sugars and only a moderate secretion of insulin.

An additional benefit of fibers is that they contain no calories, act as a broom sweeping through your intestines and slow down digestion. The health benefits include a reduced risk for developing obesity, diabetes, heart diseases and disorders of the gastrointestinal tract.

The easiest way to find food that contains complex carbohydrates is by choosing food that is high in fiber. The common recommendation for men is to consume 38 grams of fiber per day and for women 25 grams.

A focus on complex carbohydrates doesn't mean that you have to avoid simple carbohydrates at all times. In some circumstances, your body has a preference or simple carbohydrates. As an example, when performing prolonged high impact physical activity, your muscles will use up the stored glycogen in about 50 minutes. In this case, new fuel is required quickly to keep them going. The fastest way to replenish the muscles with new fuel is through consuming simple carbohydrates as it takes too much time to digest complex carbohydrates.

You will read more about this topic in the fourth circle of healthy nutrition, covering the importance of balancing the intake of food and fluid with the type and level of physical activity.

Sources of Complex Carbohydrates. Vegetables, Legumes and Fruit.

The difference between vegetables and legumes is that the latter represents the seeds of a plant and that the former comes from the plant parts like leaves, roots and stems.

All vegetables and legumes are sources of complex carbohydrates, vitamins, minerals, fibers, water and anti-oxidants. Common examples of vegetables are sweet potato, potato, broccoli, Brussels sprouts, cabbage, cucumber, kale, garlic, leafy greens, peppers, parsley, onion, eggplant, zucchini, radish and pumpkin.

Fill your plate for two-third of a variety of vegetables every day and you can feel assured that you covered the needs of your body.

There are two groups of vegetables that deserve extra attention.

The first group is cruciferous vegetables. These vegetables are known for being twice as powerful as other pant food when it comes to health benefits.

Cruciferous vegetables are broccoli, cauliflower, bok choy, cabbage, Brussels sprouts, kale, collard greens and celery.

The second group is root vegetables. What sets these vegetables apart from the other vegetables is that they grow underground with the consequence that they are higher in starches or sugars than other vegetables.

Examples of root vegetables are potato, sweet potato, yam, carrots, beet, parsnip, turnip and rutabaga.

Examples of legumes are lentils, peas, chickpeas, beans, peanuts and alfafa.

Fruit is also a great source of carbohydrates. Some fruit is higher in fructose than other but that is no reason to avoid them. Since fruit producers have done a lot the past decades to make fruit sweeter, it is good to limit yourself to 2 to 3 servings a day. 1 serving equals a medium sized apple. Also, to stimulate your body to use up the glucose and the fructose in fruit before your next meal or snack, do not combine eating fruit with other food.

Examples are apple, citrus, pineapple, pear, plum, melon, peach, grape, berries, apricot, cherry, avocado, tomato and olive.

The fruit that deserves extra attention are those high in anti-oxidants. The function of anti-oxidants is to neutralize so called free radicals, atoms or molecules formed as a result of pollution and normal body functions that require oxygen. The problem with free radicals is that they compromise the proper function of cells.

Examples of fruit that is high in anti-oxidants are blueberries, blackberries, strawberries, raspberries, prunes, plums, oranges, grapes, raisins, cherries and pomegranates.

Protein

The next calorie-containing nutrient from which the body derives energy is protein.

Protein is used mainly for building, maintaining, repairing body tissue and the production of enzymes and hormones. Protein contributes under normal circumstances to about 3 percent of the energy requirements of the body but this can increase to about 15 percent to overcome or survive extreme conditions.

Amino Acids - The Building Blocks of the Body

Digestive enzymes break down proteins into amino acids, the building blocks for body tissue and cells varying from organs to blood cells.

The building, maintaining or repairing of body tissue is a form of storing. The body can reverse this process by breaking down body tissue, mostly muscle, for energy. Another form of storage is the amino acid pool which is a short-term protein store used as a buffer for daily variations in protein intake.

Neither of the two forms of storages are meant to provide a long-term store for future needs. Taking in more protein than your body needs activates the deamination process in the liver. In this process, the liver converts the amino acids into other molecules like glucose to use as fuel or store as fat.

The human body requires 20 types of amino acids, of which 10 are essential. Essential means that your body needs to obtain them from the food you consume because it is unable to produce those amino acids itself.

The 10 essential amino acids are leucine, isoleucine, lysine, methionine, phenylalanine, threonine, tryptophan, valine, histidine and, in fact semi-essential, arginine.

The non-essential amino acids are alanine, asparagine, aspartate, cysteine, glutamate, glutamine, glycine, proline, serine and tyrosine.

Proteins from animal sources are complete proteins because they contain all 20 amino acids.

Most plant based proteins lack one or more of the essential amino acids and are therefore called incomplete proteins. Examples of plant based proteins that are sources of complete proteins are hemp, buckwheat, quinoa, chia, amaranth, sprouted lentils and soy.

If you are deficient in essential amino acids, your body has no other choice but to break down muscle tissue in order to obtain the necessary amino acids. It is therefore important that your meals contain all the essential amino acids. If you don't want to eat protein from animal sources such as meat, eggs, dairy products and fish, you can still get all the essential amino acids by consuming a variety of vegetables with beans and wild rice, lentils with wild rice, nuts and seeds.

How Much Protein Should You Eat?

Especially after the age of 50, consuming enough protein is important as the body becomes less efficient in using protein for creating muscle tissue.

This doesn't mean that to be sure you get enough you can eat extra or excessive amounts of this nutrient. There are drawbacks to eating too much protein. Balancing your protein intake is important.

Eating more protein than your body needs leads to fat storage in the first place. The liver converts any surplus of protein into sugar and then into fat. Keep in mind that elevated sugar levels also feed yeast and bacteria that can negatively affect our health.

Converting amino acids into sugar is known as the deamination process. During this process the liver removes the nitrogen molecules and releases them into the blood stream. It is then up to the kidneys to filter the nitrogen out of the blood stream and remove them from the body. This is extra work for liver and kidneys that can be avoided. Another way nitrogen molecules can leave the body is through perspiration.

Excessive protein can also stimulate the mammalian target of rapamycin (mTOR) pathway. Don't pay too much attention to these tongue-twisting words. What is essential to know is that the mTOR pathway is a biochemical process that plays a major role in the development of many cancers.

The best advice I can give to minimize the risk that this dangerous pathway becomes activated is to stop eating the refined sugars so often present in convenience or fast food. As I mentioned before, consuming more sugar than your body needs already has devastating effects on your body. Combining excessive sugar intake with eating more protein than your body requires makes things even worse.

Studies indicate that plant-based protein doesn't activate and even reverses the biochemical processes responsible for developing cancer growth. In other words, make a deliberate choice to reduce or better stop consuming protein from animals, especially when living a sedentary lifestyle.

How to figure out how much protein is right for you?

The basic rule is that most adults need about one gram of protein per kilogram of LEAN body mass, or 0.5 gram of protein per pound of lean body mass per day.

To find out what your lean body mass is you have to subtract the fat you carry with you from your total body weight. One method to find out how much body fat you have is to compare yourself with the images you can find on the internet when you search for body fat percentage pictures comparison.

Another way find out how much of your body weight is fat tissue is to step on a scale that measures your body composition, giving you beside your weight also the numbers for water content, bone mass, muscle tissue and fat tissue.

The simple math goes like this:

Body weight in pounds minus fat content in pounds times 0.5 gram = total grams of protein recommended.

As an example, if your body weight is 185 pounds of which 35 pounds is fat tissue, the recommended protein intake per day would be (185 - 35) x 0.5= 75 grams.

This basic rule works for most people. Only if you exercise frequently and aggressively you could increase your protein consumption toward the 0.75 grams per pound lean body mass.

Buy high quality proteins. When buying animal based protein, choose grass fed and avoid meats or dairy contaminated with antibiotics and hormones and fish from farms. When buying plant based protein, avoid conventionally grown and genetically modified.

Also be sure to combine eating sufficient amounts of protein with types of meaningful physical activity. Eating protein alone won't help you maintain and build muscle tissue, you need to keep working your muscles against meaningful resistance in order to stimulate your body to maintain and build muscle tissue and strengthen your joints, tendons, ligaments and bones at the same time.

Protein as Fuel for Muscles

The liver can convert amino acids, mainly from muscle tissue, into fuel for the remaining working muscles in the event that carbohydrates are not available and the body needs energy at a faster rate than can be generated from fat. This is an unwanted situation that needs to be avoided at all times since muscle tissue, the center point of good health, is so easy to lose and so hard to gain. Therefore, protecting your muscles must always have your focus.

Sources of Protein

Meats	Seafood	Dairy	Raw Nuts	Plant based
Beef	Salmon	Milk	Walnuts	Tofu
Pork	Tuna	Yogurt	Almonds	Tempeh
Lamb	Sardine	Cheese	Cashew	Lentils
Chicken	Herring	Eggs	Pecan	Beans
Turkey	Mussel	Pistachio	Quinoa	
Duck	Anchovy	Coconut	Amaranth	
Fowl	Clam	Chestnut	Chia seeds	
Wild game	Crab	Pumpkin	Hemp seeds	
Organ Meats	Lobster	Sesame	Buckwheat	
Mackerel	Sunflower	Soy		
Oyster	Macademia	Spirulina		
	Scallop			
	Shrimp			
	Squid			

Fat

Fat is an important macronutrient. In fact, we can't live without it. Fat is necessary for a host of bodily functions.

What has given dietary fat a bad name is the idea that it makes you fat because it contains 9 calories per gram. However, unlike the sugar from carbohydrates, dietary fat doesn't influence your insulin levels. This means that your body can stay in the fat burning mode described earlier.

Fat increases the feeling of satiety for a longer time than does carbohydrate. You will probably consume fewer calories from fat than you would from carbohydrates in order to maintain the same feeling of satiety. About 35 percent of the calories we take in should come from fat.

Fat and the Function of Insulin

The fat we consume is broken down during the digestive process into small particles called fatty acids and used as fuel throughout the day. They are small enough to flow in and out the fat cells through the cell membranes and are the main source of energy for daily low to medium impact activities.

This flow in and out of the fat cells stops as soon as you eat food that increases your blood glucose and subsequently your insulin levels. Remember that high blood glucose levels are toxic to the body. Insulin therefore immediately locks up the release of fatty acids, carbohydrates and protein from the body cells to ensure that the body uses up the glucose in the blood stream first. Fatty acids, bundled in groups of three and stored as triglycerides, are unable to flow through the cell membranes.

The release of other hormones and enzymes is required to convert the triglycerides back into fatty acids, a process that can only take place when insulin level is normal.

Types of Fat

Trans fats are fats to avoid at all times. During a process called hydrogenation, liquid fats are changed into solid fats to make it easier to use them in baked goods, margarines, chips, salads, and breakfast cereals. This type of fat is detrimental to the body, even in small amounts. Read food labels and ingredient lists carefully and put the item back on the shelf whenever you read the following words: trans fats, partially hydrogenated fats, vegetable shortening, or margarine.

Saturated fats, solid at room temperature, have a bad name too but don't deserve this as saturated fat is important for heart, lungs, bones, hormones, immune system, cell membranes, liver, skin, taste and the feeling of satiety.

Meat and dairy products are common animal sources of saturated fat while coconut oil and red palm oil are plant-based sources. Saturated fat remains stable when heated, whereas unsaturated fat, especially polyunsaturated fat from corn, safflower, sunflower, canola, soybean and cottonseed oil, easily oxidizes and forms free radicals that damage body cells.

Mono- and polyunsaturated fat are liquid at room temperature. The difference between monounsaturated and polyunsaturated fats lies in their chemical structure. The former has one double bond between the carbon atoms in the carbon chain backbone, whereas the latter has two.

Polyunsaturated fat is more solid than monounsaturated fat but less solid than saturated fat. Both fats are healthy and therefore important ingredients of the meals we consume.

Sources of monounsaturated fat are olive oil, avocados, nuts and seeds.

Polyunsaturated fat can be broken down into the essential fatty acids omega-3 and omega-6. The term essential means that the body can obtain them only through food intake.

One difference between omega-3 and omega-6 fatty acids is that they have opposite effects. Those from omega-6 fatty acids tend to increase inflammation, an important component of the immune response, blood clotting, and cell proliferation, whereas those from omega-3 fatty acids decrease those functions.

Balance between the two is crucial to maintain optimum health. Consuming more omega-6 fatty acids than omega-3 fatty acids sets off the production of cytokines by cell membranes. Cytokines are chemicals that cause inflammatory responses in the body.

The problem with the typical North American diet is that it contains 14 to 25 times more omega-6 than omega-3 fatty acids, whereas most experts agree that the optimal omega-6 to 3 ratio should range from 1:1 to 4:1. This dietary imbalance causes inflammation in the body and is believed to be partly responsible for the rise in chronic diseases such as asthma, heart diseases, cancers and autoimmune diseases. The lack of balance between omega-3 and omega-6 fatty acids is also linked to obesity, depression, hyperactivity and even violence.

Therefore, choose polyunsaturated fat high in omega-3 fatty acids when preparing meals.

Good sources of omega-3 fatty acids are dark green leafy vegetables, walnuts, kiwi, krill oil and fish such as wild caught salmon, halibut, sardines, light chunk tuna, catfish, cod, albacore, trout, herring and clams, all wild caught.

Food rich in omega-6 fatty acids are vegetable oils like corn, safflower, sunflower, soybean and cottonseed oil.

Cholesterol

Although feared by many people for its link to heart diseases, cholesterol is essential for the production hormones, healthy cell walls, bile acids to aid in fat digestion and vitamin D.

The liver makes about 80 percent of the cholesterol we need and the rest comes from the food we eat. The liver decreases the production of cholesterol when we increase our fat intake and increases the production of cholesterol when we decrease our fat intake.

Cholesterol is Not the Cause of Heart Diseases

For a long time, cholesterol was thought to be the main cause of heart disease, but research has shown that the lipoprotein, see below, that carries the cholesterol is the actual culprit.

Causes of heart diseases are:

High levels of triglycerides as a result of eating refined carbohydrates, as in many convenience, fast and processed food,

High levels of low-density lipoproteins (LDL), also known as bad cholesterol as a result of eating refined carbohydrates,

Low levels of high-density lipoproteins (HDL), also known as good cholesterol as a result of eating refined carbohydrates.

The understanding that cholesterol is not the actual cause of heart disease is slowly but steadily gaining more ground. It is worth mentioning that the U.S. Dietary Guidelines Advisory Committee announced on 07 January 2016 in its 2015 – 2020 dietary guidelines that "cholesterol is not considered a nutrient of concern for overconsumption."

You can read the dietary guidelines for Americans on to the website http://health.gov/dietaryguidelines/2015/guidelines

Cholesterol is considered good or bad depending on whether it is carried through the bloodstream by HDL or LDL.

Inflammation of the walls of the arteries and veins is often a result of prolonged increase in blood glucose and insulin. To repair the inflammation, LDL present in the blood stream is used to mortar up the damaged areas.

Low HDL levels and high LDL levels are not the cause but a symptom of cardiovascular disease and therefore a marker of the body's inflammatory state.

This is why it is important to learn about your total cholesterol in relation with HDL, LDL and triglycerides, and not just about your total cholesterol.

Total Cholesterol, HDL, LDL and Triglycerides, Important Ratios

Values are provided in mg/dl in the US or in mmol/L in Australia, Canada and most European countries.

mg/dl = milligram per liter
mmol/L= millimole per liter
100 mg/dl = 2.586 mmol/l

General guidelines for desirable amounts are:
total cholesterol
less than 200 mg/dL or 5.17 mmol/L

high density lipoprotein (HDL)
greater than 60mg/dL or 1.55 mmol/L

low density lipoprotein (LDL)
less than 100 mg/dL or 2.59 mmol/L

triglycerides
less than 150 mg/dL or 1.69 mmol/L

Aside from the individual numbers, ratios are important as well. The optimal total cholesterol/HDL cholesterol should be below 3.5 and the triglyceride/HDL ratio should be below 2.

These numbers are indications. Consult your doctor to learn how the levels and ratios relate to your specific situation.

High blood sugar as a result from eating carbohydrates not only leads to low HDL and high LDL levels but also makes LDL particles small and dense which accelerates the build-up of plaque deposits in the arteries.

Eating good fats such as olive oil, avocados, nuts and seeds, coconut oil and butter from grass fed cows leads to the opposite effect or high HDL levels and low LDL levels. In addition, the LDL particles become larger and fluffier which makes it more difficult for these particles to stick to the artery walls.

Food on your daily menu that is low in fat and high in refined carbohydrates leads to low HDL, high triglycerides, high LDL and small and dense LDL particles.

A more healthy practice is to consume food that is high in good fats and low in refined carbohydrates leading to high levels of HDL, low triglycerides, low LDL and larger and fluffier LDL particles.

Improving the ratios mentioned above by focusing on the symptoms is what medication does. Taking away what causes the inflammation in the first place is the proper way to deal with ratios that are out of balance. It is good to realize that just like refined carbohydrates cause inflammation, stress and environmental factors like second hand cigarette smoke and toxins can be equally damaging.

Reducing the consumption of food and drinks that are high in sugar together with reducing stress and keeping your environment clean are important steps to restore normal cholesterol levels.

Micro Nutrients and the Role of Enzymes

Vitamins and minerals are called micronutrients. They don't contain calories but are important for all sorts of chemical reactions in the body. Water is also a micronutrient although many people prefer to call it a macronutrient because of the volume we consume compared to the other nutrients. Your body obviously doesn't care and simply considers water the most important nutrient.

Vitamins

Vitamins have always had a mysterious aura with magical powers. Many people are willing to pay a lot of money for vitamin supplements.

Supplements can't do or be more than what they are, supplements. Your body's needs should be met through healthy eating. You can't repair poor eating habits with supplements.

Maximize vitamin intake through eating a variety of colourful fruit and vegetables, preferably those that are in season. Because many vitamins are lost or destroyed during cooking, avoid overcooking and keep your vegetables a bit crunchy.

If you feel you are deficient in certain vitamins, look for ways to adjust your food intake and have yourself checked for any kind of vitamin deficiency.

Vitamins are categorized in two groups, water-soluble and fat-soluble. The fat-soluble vitamins, A, D, E and K, are absorbed with fat and are stored in the body. In contrast, water-soluble vitamins, vitamin B complex and C, cannot be stored. The kidneys secrete them when you take in more than you need. This difference is important: taking in too much of the water-soluble vitamins is pointless and storing too much of the fat-soluble vitamins could cause negative effects to the body.

The Most Important Vitamins - their Functions and Sources

Vitamin	Function	Found In
B1 (Thiamin)	carbohydrate metabolism, Nervous system	whole grains, nuts, legumes
B2 (Riboflavin)	protein metabolism, energy metabolism, skin- and eye health	whole grains, nuts, eggs, dark green leafy vegetables
B3 (Niacin)	energy metabolism (glycolysis *), fat synthesis	whole grains, nuts, eggs, turkey, chicken, fish
B5 (Pantothenic acid)	energy metabolism, (gluconeogenesis **)	all non-processed food

B6 (Pyridoxine)	fat metabolism, protein metabolism, glycolysis	whole grains, eggs, meats
B12 (Cobalamine)	fat metabolism, protein metabolism, glycolysis	eggs, meat, poultry
C (Ascorbic acid)	collagen formation and iron absorption	fresh fruit and vegetables
A (Retinol)	skin/eye health, immune system, cell health	butter, cheese, liver, egg-yolks, pigmented fruit and vegetables
D3 (Calciferol)	skin/eye health, absorption of calcium and phosphorus	sun, fish, liver oil and eggs
E (Tocopherol)	antioxidant	vegetable oils and eggs
K	bone strength, blood clot development	dark green leafy vegetables, intestinal bacteria.
H (Biotin)	gluconeogenesis, glucose and fatty acid synthesis	egg yolks, dark green leafy vegetables.
Folic acid	red blood cell synthesis, foetal development	whole grains, green leafy vegetables, beans, oranges, bananas.

* Glycolysis = the breakdown of glucose into chemical compound cells use to create energy.

** Gluconeogenesis = the conversion of non-carbohydrate sources into glucose by the liver.

Minerals and their Functions

The roll of minerals is to activate a variety of enzyme reactions. Some examples of minerals and their functions;

Mineral	Function
Calcium	bones and teeth, muscle contraction, heart and nerve function and blood clotting
Magnesium	muscles, bones, liver, muscle/nerve function
Potassium	heart rhythm, nerve function, cell building
Sodium	regulating body fluid and nerve function
Manganese	carbohydrate and protein metabolism, vitamin B1 utilization, connective and nerve tissue
Zinc	carbohydrate metabolism, wound healing, sexual function, protein synthesis
Iron	haemoglobin formation, oxygen transportation
Phosphorus	bones and teeth, calcium absorption, energy production and cell membranes
Chromium	heart, insulin activity, glucose utilization, cholesterol utilization
Copper	production of haemoglobin, utilization of cholesterol, formation of elastic tissue
Silicon	bone, collagen and cartilage formation and elastic tissue.
Boron	reduces loss of calcium
Tin	growth and protein synthesizing
Vanadium	bones and teeth, lowers blood lipids and inhibits cholesterol synthesis.

Balance is King

Minerals work in balance with one another as well as with vitamins and the macronutrients carbohydrate, protein and fat. Too much of one could cause a chain reaction of deficiencies in others. For example:

Too much	Leads to
Calcium	Loss of magnesium and zinc
Sodium and potassium	Deficiency of calcium and magnesium
Calcium and magnesium	Deficiency of sodium and potassium
Potassium	Loss of sodium
Sodium	Loss of potassium
Copper	Loss of zinc
Zinc	Loss of copper and iron
Phosphorus	Loss of calcium

Water

Water is the most important nutrient and accounts for about 60 percent of your body mass. Lean body tissues such as muscle, heart and liver contain about 75 percent water, whereas fat contains about 10 to 20 percent water.

Water is crucial for the transport of glucose, oxygen and fats to working muscles, elimination of waste products, heat absorption from working muscles, regulation of body temperature, lubrication of joints and cushioning organs and tissues.

Staying hydrated is important for optimal performance and smooth functioning of body systems. It takes only a 2 percent loss of body weight through losing body fluid for performance to suffer.

How do you measure your hydration status?

Thirst is the most obvious sign that you need to drink, but not the best sign because when you experience thirst, you are already mildly dehydrated.

Drinking a certain amount of water every day is one way to maintain an adequate level of hydration but this method loses its accuracy when external conditions such as temperature, humidity and physical activity change.

The easiest way to measure your hydration status is through checking the color of your urine. Pale and plenty is a good sign of hydration whereas dark and scant indicates the opposite. Keep in mind that vitamin supplements can give urine a darker color. Go by volume if this is the case.

Signs of dehydration are muscle cramps, reduced performance, weakness, fatigue, headache, nausea and dizziness, confusion and irrational behavior.

Tips to help you stay hydrated are having a water bottle with you during your workouts sessions, drinking regularly throughout the day and drinking cold water as it rehydrates the body more effectively than warm water. Sports drinks are not a good choice since they are high in sugar, which is unnecessary for activities that last less than 60 minutes.

The Role of Enzymes

Enzymes control all the chemical reactions in the body. Without enzymes your body can't utilize the nutrients, vitamins, minerals and hormones for metabolic work.

An example of an enzyme is amylase present in saliva, needed to convert carbohydrates into glucose.

Other chemical reactions controlled by enzymes are the building of body tissue, storage of food, the removal of carbon dioxide from the lungs and waste from the blood, the conversion of protein into sugar or fat and the conversion of carbohydrates into fat.

Whatever biochemical process occurs in your body, enzymes play a key role.

Enzymes are made of amino acids, the building blocks created from the digestion of protein or the breakdown of muscle tissue. Hundreds of amino acids are strung together in a specific order to carry out specific chemical reactions.

Each organ and tissue has its own particular enzymes to perform specialized metabolic work.

Enzymes are created by the body. The pancreas and small intestine produce digestive enzymes.

Raw food contains many enzymes and it is here where a serious controversy begins between advocates of eating raw food and those who say that it is best to mainly eat cooked food.

Advocates of eating raw food say that it is an important component of our daily meals because of the enzymes they contain. The more enzymes we obtain from raw food the fewer enzymes the body has to produce itself.

Why raw food? The answer is that enzymes are destroyed when food is heated over 118 degree Fahrenheit or 48 degree Celcius.

Those who say that you better cook your food don't fall for this argument and say that the enzymes in plants are only there to serve the plants and not humans.

After being ingested, the enzymes in plants do not function as replacements for human digestive enzymes. The plant enzymes get digested by our own digestive juices along with the rest of of the food and are absorbed and utilized as nutrients.

Although they agree that plant enzymes can be useful to maximize health, they say that it is not true that eating raw food requires less enzyme production from your body, and that plant enzymes don't aid in their own digestion inside the human body.

The supporters of eating raw food have a point when they say that cooking, and especially baking and frying, not only destroys the enzymes but also many other nutrients in food such as vitamins.

This is without doubt true. Comparing raw broccoli to cooked broccoli, about 25 percent of the vitamin C and about 20 percent of the selenium is lost during cooking. At the same time, other nutrients in broccoli hardly change.

On the other hand, the benefit of cooking is that it destroys some of the harmful anti-nutrients in raw food which increases absorption of healthy nutrients. Cooking or steaming vegetables also breaks down and alters cell structures so that fewer enzymes are needed to digest the food, instead of more.

Studies made clear that the antioxidant activity of cooked tomatoes is much higher than from uncooked tomatoes.

Be careful though with baking food. When food is baked, especially fried or barbecued, at high temperatures, toxic compounds such as acrylamide is formed. This won't happen when food is boiled or steamed.

In short, there is a place for raw and cooked food and we should have both on our menu on a daily basis.

We humans don't have the digestive system of plant eaters to live on raw food only but it is better equipped than the digestive system of meat eaters.

And that may be the answer that comes closest to the truth, go for the best of both worlds.

Choose for a sufficient quantity of raw fruit, vegetables, nuts and seeds as well as for cooked vegetables since they too provide your body with the essential healthy nutrients. Just don't overcook your veggies.

As always, choose as often as you can for organically produced vegetables and fruit and avoid processed food.

The Second Circle of Healthy Nutrition, Quantity

Knowing what types of food are best for the body and which to avoid is a vital step toward healthy eating. Having said that, no matter how good the quality of your diet, eating and drinking more than your body needs inevitably leads to health problems.

Taste and Comfort

Our digestive system doesn't care at all about the presentation of our meals or even about taste. The only thing it is interested in and searches for are the 6 macro- and micronutrients to keep our body systems going. The digestive system dismantles the meals we consume, picks out what it needs and stores or disposes of the rest.

When humans lived as hunters and gatherers, they used their 5 senses to determine whether they could eat something or needed to avoid it. Taste has always been the final gatekeeper that gives a green light when the taste is right and feels good and a red light if the taste was wrong. Although not water-proof, this system has been good enough to help us survive for thousands of generations.

In the natural quest to enhance our feelings of safety, comfort and convenience, creating food that tastes good and makes us feel good became important. As mentioned before, it is the reward center in our brainstem, part of the reptilian brain, which stimulates this behaviour.

This center makes very strong demands and never seems to get enough. Succumbing to the demands of the reward centre is easy and can make one forget about the needs of the rest of the body, which may differ from those of the reward center.

Thus, we have evolved over the last 6 or 7 generations from eating what Mother Earth provided, to eating our present day diets in quantities that have created the health problems many of us are now dealing with.

Your Body Can't Help It

Our body loves energy coming in but hates energy going out and this is what has enabled humankind to survive up until today. Sadly, it is this same basic formula that is responsible for the premature death of millions in developed countries today.

When humans lived as hunters and gatherers, it was never certain when the next meal would show up. Days of abundance in food supply could change at any moment into a period of famine. The only way humankind could overcome those periods of famine was to have a built-in body system that would store part of the incoming energy in times of abundance for later use.

The conditions in which we live may have changed, but our bodies haven't. They are still functioning the way they were wired and operating for thousands of years, always preserve and never waste.

The Defense Mechanisms of Your Body

Anything out of the normal state of affairs equals stress for the body. Whether the stress is caused by famine, draught, illness, grief, strenuous labor, fight or flight, all these states have one thing in common, they require more energy than during normal conditions.

As soon as the human body senses stress, it sets off the secretion of the hormone cortisol, also known as the stress-hormone. This hormone signals code red for the body, sending out the warning to hold on to every calorie as it may be needed to withstand whatever is attacking the body.

This is another reason why diets rarely work. The moment you start a diet, your body senses stress, shifts into stress mode and begins to activate mechanisms to conserve calories, the exact opposite of what you are trying to achieve. You'll read more about how stress affects your body and well-being in the "Mastering Your Eating Habits".

"But I lost 7 pounds in two weeks. Doesn't that mean something?"

The answer to this question is yes and no at the same time. One of the effects of reducing your overall food intake is that you also reduce the intake of carbohydrates. As each molecule of this nutrient is stored in the body with three molecules of water, the greater part of your weight loss is caused by the loss of water. When you reach the point where you cannot reduce your food intake, and therefore carbohydrate intake any further, weight loss slows down or comes to a standstill.

Counting Calories and Servings

Respecting the way the body works and what it is capable of is the foundation for everything you would like your body to do. Your body is a tool, a vehicle that executes the ideas and actions developed by your mind. The point is that what is feasible by your mind's standard isn't always feasible for the body.

A simple example could be your idea about moving a heavy box. You may think that you can lift it but when your body is lacking the strength, it simply will not happen. The same goes for weight loss. You may come up with the plan to lose 3 pounds of body fat every week but if that is too much for your body to handle it will not cooperate.

Restoring Balance

We can't leave it to the reward centre in our brainstem to decide what and how much we can or must eat and drink. The rest of our body has its demands too. The two aspects of the wellness wheel that play a role here are mental/emotional and physical health. It is important to consider the demands of both when we eat and drink. Balance is the key and is what we must strive toward by consciously using our conscious mind.

Many people have tried tools such as calorie counters and serving counters to restore balance and control their eating and drinking behaviours. Although helpful, the disadvantage of this rational approach is that it has no connection with emotions and feelings.

Using calorie and serving counters makes sense when you consider that we can convert the energy of all what we eat and drink into calories. It looks like a sound and simple system that can't fail. A pound of body fat equals 3,500 calories. As long as you take in 500 calories per day less than you used to, you will lose one pound of body fat per week. Do this consistently and let time do its work. Problem solved. True on paper, but reality shows that it works only for a happy few. The majority of people struggling to lose weight apparently need more than this simple tool.

A key reason for this is that, aside from the fact that calorie in calorie out is a myth as described earlier, most people find counting calories and servings to be an impractical and tedious job, even when using apps on mobile devices. Another reason is that a clear directive about the number of calories permitted per day isn't enough by itself to ignite the perseverance needed to eat less.

The fact that 95 to 98 percent of the people who attempt to lose weight fail repeatedly, is clear evidence of how difficult it is to control eating habits. How then can you deal with the temptation to eat more than your body needs and being unable to hold yourself back?

Mindful Eating and Drinking

Sustainable weight loss begins with understanding and respecting the functions and systems of body and mind. Once that has been established, one can begin making the changes that will set off the desired effects without having to deal with unwanted side effects such as loss of motivation or stress.

In the first circle of healthy nutrition, "Quality", I covered the importance of eating the type of food your body needs to function well. "Quantity" is about creating the right mindset to recognize the signals of your body telling you that you've had enough and that eating more isn't needed or beneficial.

Keep it Simple and Effective

Your brain is the only tool that is effective, geared to your specific needs, always at hand and works flawlessly if you know how to use it. We don't need factors outside our body such as calorie counters and serving counters in order to control our food intake. Everything we need is present in our body. The art is to create the conditions that enable you to detect its signals.

Below are 10 simple and effective strategies for mindful eating and drinking to replace the calorie and serving counting practices. The strategies look at eating and drinking from the bodies' perspective, meant to nourish your body as a whole, physically as well as mentally and emotionally.

When reading through the list you may feel thoughts come up such as "makes sense, that's new, didn't know that and that sounds a bit extreme". Accept these thoughts for now and keep an open mind. No need to answer the question at this moment whether or not you can or will be able to apply the strategies.

Thinking and talking about them is enough. Gently move judgements away.

10 Simple and Effective Strategies for Mindful Eating and Drinking

1. Eat from a 9-inch plate. Plates and portion sizes have become bigger and bigger over the years and we tend to continue eating as long as there is food on the plate. A 9-inch plate is the first tool to limit the amount of food we eat.

2. Eat about 20 percent less than you usually do.

3. Make eating the only activity you engage in when you eat. In other words, don't combine eating with watching television, reading or other activities. If you combine eating with other activities, you're not eating consciously, in other words mindless, and run the risk that you'll have finished your plate before you know it resulting in feeling unsatisfied and refilling your plate.

4. Don't drink when you eat. The function of digestive enzymes is to break down the nutrients we consume. Fluid dilutes the digestive enzymes making them less effective.

5. Don't put the serving dishes on the table. Keeping these out of sight makes it easier stop at one helping.

6. Lay your fork down after every bite. A step up is to close your eyes, feel the food in your mouth and focus on chewing. Take your time to taste the food and distinguish a sweet, bitter or salty taste.

7. About 20 minutes from the moment you begin eating, your stomach secretes a hormone called leptin to signal your brain that you are satisfied and that you can stop eating. Slow and conscious eating not only enables the digestive enzymes to do their work but also gives leptin the chance to reach your brain, and your brain to pick up the signal.

8. Oxygen is as fundamental to a meal as the food itself. Eating is similar to any other type of physical activity in the sense that it is an aerobic action and therefore requires oxygen.

Slowing down breathing before eating and maintaining slow and deep breathing, meaning breathing from you belly, during and after eating oxygenates the digestive organs. It also promotes parasympathetic dominance, endorphin release and the feeling of relaxation and well-being, which in turn promotes effective digestion, assimilation and calorie burning.

Eating while in a stressful state on the other hand promotes sympathetic dominance and changes your breathing pattern into shallow and high. The consequence is that your digestion will slow down and that the food will stay longer in your gut. As covered before, stress negatively affects the number of healthy gut bacteria, in turn affecting brain function and the quality of the intestinal lining. What could happen next is that bacteria and particles that should have stayed in your intestines enter the bloodstream and set off a wide range of health effects.

Therefore, avoid eating in a stressful state. Lower your stress levels by concentrating on slow and deep breathing to promote relaxation. If you eat alone, avoid stressful thoughts. Think of something pleasurable instead and focus on the food you eat. When you eat with other people, have conversations that keep the atmosphere relaxed and have some music playing in the background that promotes relaxation.

9. Keep a food and fluid journal for a week or two. Most people don't like keeping a food and fluid journal because they think that it is not effective. The opposite is true. This journal is not meant to count calories or servings, but to write down what and when you eat and drink. No long stories, unless you want to. Quick, short notes will do.

10. Practice daily the technique of prolonged pointed attention with vivid creative imagination which we will cover further in this part of the book.

Studies have shown that food and fluid journals are powerful tools for losing weight. In fact, people who keep a food and fluid journal lose about twice as much weight as people who don't, a clear fact that speaks for itself.

A food and fluid journal works for three important reasons,

It creates awareness and holds you accountable. You have to write down everything you eat and drink. It helps you to think twice about why and what you eat.

It provides clarity. Looking at your food and drink intake during the day makes clear in an instant where you can make better choices.

It supports you. It helps you to stay on track during difficult days. Reading through your journal and seeing what you have achieved gives your self-esteem a boost and helps you to persevere.

A Food and Fluid Journal

What should a food and fluid journal look like?

There are no real rules here. You can use online tools but a pen and a blank sheet of paper work just as well. It's important that you have the journal at hand every time you eat and/or drink. A simple and straight forward food and fluid journal looks like the diagram below.

Food and Fluid Journal   **Week #.............**

Meal	Monday	Tuesday	Wednesday	Thursday	Friday	Saturday	Sunday
Breakfast							
Snack							
Lunch							
Snack							
Dinner							
Snack							

Record only what you eat and drink. There is no need to count calories or servings because that is not very effective and it makes keeping a food journal tedious. What sense does it make to force your body into a restricted calorie intake when your physical activity varies from day to day? Again, it is all about balance.

When you mindfully eat small meals or snacks and eat just enough that you don't feel hungry, you can't go wrong. Learn to listen to your body. Sometimes you need to eat extra and sometimes you can do with less.

Learning to listen to your body is also important to decipher real eating from emotional eating. Whenever you feel you want to eat or drink, take the time to ask yourself why you want to eat. Is it because you are hungry or because you feel tired, bored, sad and so on?

Create a routine of:

Focus - Action - Reflection

Review your food log at the end of each week and see where you can make adjustments in quality and quantity. Make small adjustments to start. It is easier to maintain small changes than big ones. Stick with every change you make. Then continue with the next week and so on.

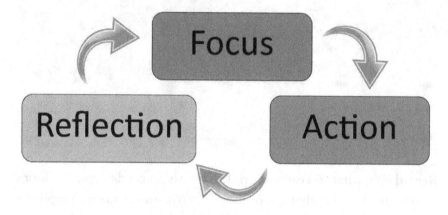

Focus-Action-Reflection

Your body will respond to every change you make. Those reactions can range from feeling good to feeling uncomfortable. Put yourself at ease and realize that your body needs time to adjust to the changes. This can take vary from days to weeks.

Your daily practice using the technique of prolonged pointed attention with vivid creative imagination which we will cover after the chapters timing and balance will help you with this.

The Third Circle Of Healthy Nutrition, Timing

Consuming good quality food and fluid in moderation is an important step toward healthy eating. The logical follow up is timing, the subject of the third circle in this guide. It covers how often and when to eat.

The Benefits of Frequent Small Meals

Seen it from your body's point of view, it needs a regular input of food and fluid to keep your internal fire, known as your metabolism, going. Compare it with a wood stove. The best way to keep the stove burning is by feeding it with small logs over regular intervals. Your metabolism works similar. Eating regular small meals guarantees a consistent smooth burning of your metabolism without the risk of overloading your body with fuel or causing it to lag because of lack of fuel.

Refraining from eating in order to lose weight is about the worst thing you can do. Remember that your body has a built-in mechanism to survive during conditions of scarcity such as those in which our ancestors lived.

Whenever their bodies sensed an interruption in food intake, they instantly shifted into starvation mode, a stress reaction to hold on to every calorie possible. While our conditions have changed, the way our body works hasn't. You can tell your body a hundred times that there is no reason to go into starvation mode and slow down metabolism, but that won't prevent your body from reacting the way it is wired.

If you want your body to behave in a certain way, you have to understand and respect its systems and treat it accordingly. Never interfere with its systems and programming.

Respecting the needs of your body means that you do what's necessary to prevent your body from moving into the stress mode. This goes further than quality and quantity and explains the importance of timing; feeding the body at regular intervals. This third essential component keeps your metabolism running without interruption.

Eating five or six small meals spread out over the day is better than eating three big meals such as breakfast, lunch and dinner. Frequent eating provides your body with an ongoing, manageable energy supply that is in line with its needs and functions. Be careful though as eating frequent small meals holds the risk that you eat more than necessary. Reduce quantity and question yourself why you want to eat. Is it because you're feeling hungry or are you trying to justify emotional eating?

To help you get into the habit of spreading your food intake throughout the day and limiting your food intake at the same time, continue to use the same food log you are using to control the quality and the quantity of your food intake.

Breakfast, Your Most Important Meal of the Day

Start the day with a good breakfast. Your body is ready to receive the nutrients and needs them to fire up your metabolism after a night of fasting. Elevated levels of the stress hormone cortisol assist in this process. Compare the working of cortisol with the choke in your car. When you start your car's cold engine in the morning, a rich air and fuel mixture gets the engine going. Cortisol is doing the same for your body. So be sure that sufficient fuel is present to fire up your internal systems.

Don't wait until snack time or lunch time thinking that you can rely on your body's fat stores. This doesn't work because your body will immediately slow down your metabolism making you feel lethargic. On top of that, research has shown that when you skip breakfast, you will more than make up the missed calories throughout the rest of the day. Consciously or unconsciously, you will eat more over the course of the day than you would have if you had started the day with a good breakfast.

Your heart also benefits from a good breakfast. During the night, your blood becomes a little sticky and breakfast helps to unstick it. Not eating a decent breakfast increases the risk of blood clotting with an ensuing higher risk for heart attacks and strokes.

Intermittent Fasting

Going from eating three big square meals per day to eating six *small* meals spread out evenly over the day guarantees a consistent smooth burning of your metabolism without the risk of overloading your body with fuel or causing it to lag because of lack of fuel.

Some people argue that our ancestors never had the luxury of six small meals and snacks spread out over the day. They ate when food was available and had no other choice than to fast during shorter or longer periods of famine. Luckily, their body was very well capable to deal with irregular availability of food. Although our body has the same capability, many people have lost this capability due to the nature of the Western diet.

Longer periods of fasting have their benefits. Studies show that fasting helps to improve insulin sensitivity which in turn leads to normalized blood sugar and insulin levels. Remember that insulin works as a key on the surface of cells allowing them to pull in glucose from the blood stream. Improved insulin sensitivity means that receptors on the outside of a cell better respond to insulin.

The better cells respond to insulin, the better they will be able to pull in glucose. The result will be that less glucose remains behind in the blood stream and the less will be converted into fatty acids and stored as body fat.

Since elevated blood sugar and insulin levels cause inflammation in the body, fasting can help reducing these levels which in turn helps with reducing inflammatory responses.

Some other benefits of fasting are that it normalizes the levels of hormones that regulate feelings of hunger, stimulates the body to tap into the fat sources for energy and significantly promotes the production of the human growth hormone (HGH).

The production of HGH begins to gradually decline around the age of 35 and is responsible for the beginning of the aging process. Fasting can raise the production of HGH which helps with slowing down the aging process and because HGH is a fat burning hormone, it also helps with weight loss.

Fasting also decreases the build-up of free radicals that cause oxidative stress and eventually speed up the aging process.

In other words, intermitted fasting can help to reset import body functions.

Intermittent fasting means committing to restricting your food intake to a specific window of time, say eight hours, for instance from noon till eight in the evening.

This implies that outside this time window you limit yourself to drinking water, tea and coffee without milk, sugar or any type of non-caloric sweetener.

Although intermittent fasting is one of the most effective methods to lose unwanted fat, it is definitely not an eating regime good for everybody. I don't recommend this method for anybody under 30, people with health conditions and during pregnancy. Use common sense and consult your doctor when in doubt.

Another reason why this eating regime is not good for everybody is that your body may not be yet ready for it.

The moment your body will be ready for this eating regime is when it has shifted from being a so called sugar burner to a fat burner.

Your body is wired to use fat as a primary source of fuel. Due to the typical Western diet which is high in refined carbohydrates, most people's metabolic systems have become lazy and adjusted to mainly relying on carbohydrates, which changed them into sugar burners.

All of a sudden depriving yourself of carbohydrate or sugar rich food while still being a sugar burner immediately leads to stress and shifts your body into starvation mode with all ensuing consequences as I set out before.

This is the reason why crash-diets don't work. Your body isn't a machine you can switch all of a sudden into a different mode. The effects of crash-diets are well known. Those who tried looked and felt terrible after a week or two, were not a pleasure to have around, eventually accepted their defeat and regained what they had lost in a matter of weeks.

This is why I recommend normalizing food intake first which begins with eating six small meals per day.

Before you can consider beginning with intermittent fasting you need to learn your body using fatty acids as primary source of fuel. This takes time and begins with changing your eating habits by replacing processed food and other easy digestible carbohydrate rich food by whole food, preferably organically grown and healthy fats as in nuts, seeds, avocados, coconut oil, olive oil and butter.

Whole food such as vegetables is dense and high in fiber. Eating this food will result in a slow release of the stored sugars, in turn leading to normalized blood glucose and insulin levels, in turn enabling your body to begin burning fat for fuel instead of metabolizing sugar and converting and storing any surplus as fat.

Varying from one to three months your metabolic system will get increasingly better at burning fat and it is at this point you can begin with postponing your breakfast every day for about an hour. Don't fear you'll feel hungry all the time. One of the effects of intermittent fasting and your changed eating pattern will be that your hunger feelings and sugar cravings will virtually have disappeared because of normalized insulin levels.

Do it when you feel ready for it. Begin with once or twice a week and gradually build up from there. Do at days that you are not too physically active. Give it time, be patient, push yourself a bit but also allow yourself setbacks and observe how your body responds. Think of the routine of Focus, Action and Reflection.

Whenever you feel the urge to eat something let it be something that won't spike your insulin, in other words no sweets or flour containing items but slow digestible carbohydrates, some protein and healthy fats.

Intermittent fasting is not a permanent eating program. Once your metabolic system has reset itself and you are at normal weight you can gradually increase your meal frequency again.

Planning Your Meals and Snacks

Feeding your body at regular intervals with the right nutrients requires planning. How can you ensure that you will always have a healthy meal or snack available, never run short on food, and never need to get fast food?

The answer is creating a weekly meal plan.

Sound difficult? Not at all! It is not rocket science. It's all about forming a routine. Pick a day of the week to plan your meals, say a Saturday afternoon. Grab a blank sheet of paper and write down what you want to eat every day of the upcoming week.

Keep it simple. Stick to two or three variations for breakfast at the beginning and do the same for your lunch and snacks.

Dinner is a little more complicated. To help you with that you'll find in this book a "7-Day Meal Plan" with meals and snacks for the entire week, together with a complete shopping list. Once you get the hang of it, you'll find it no problem to compose healthy meals yourself or select them from sources such as magazines or the internet.

Shopping

Once you have planned your meals and snacks for the week, it is time to prepare for shopping. Below are some tips for efficient shopping.

Keep a blank sheet of paper and a pen at a designated spot in the kitchen and write down every day the items that are running low. This way you minimize the chance that you will forget something while shopping and it saves the time and money of extra trips to the supermarket for those forgotten items.

On your shopping day, complete the list by adding the items for your meals and snacks together with all the other things you need. The best day to do your errands is on a Tuesday as this is the least crowded day of the week.

When you make your shopping list, group the items to match the route you will be following through your supermarket. This makes shopping much more efficient as the items on your list will be in the same order as you will find them in your supermarket.

Almost all supermarkets are designed the same way.

On entering the store you'll find flowers and plants. They look and smell pretty and give a fresh impression.

Produce and fruit are next. They look cool, crisp and pure and stimulate the experience of fresh and healthy which is what people like to connect to.

After produce and fruit comes the bakery with the comforting and inviting smell of bread and related products. The smell is meant to make you hungry.

The bakery is often followed up by an area where food and non-food items are promoted with deals such as buy one get two or half price.

Next is the pharmacy together with the health and beauty aisles. Drop off your prescriptions and come back later. Don't wait and hang around as you may be tempted to buy something you don't really need.

The ends of the aisles always get extra attention. That's where you can find new products or products that have a relation with a time of the year or a special event.

The inner aisles are mostly for processed food items. Be sure to stick to your grocery list here.

Dairy products, eggs and meat are always located at the far back end of the store. These products are essential for most people, forcing them to cross the entire store and pass along everything else the store has to offer.

Don't go shopping on an empty stomach. The temptation to buy unhealthy snacks is too high. It will be harder to concentrate on the shopping list which puts you at risk for making poor decisions or forgetting things.

Keep a spot in your bag or pocket for a calculator and a magnifier to help you read the labels and ingredient lists and quickly figure out the best deal per pound or gram.

Focus on whole food in the outer aisles as they are generally healthier and cheaper. Buy in bulk when possible and pay attention to ads offering special deals and coupons.

When you are in the inner aisles, remember that the highest priced products are placed at eye level. Look at the lower or higher shelves for lower-priced products. Know that the products kids like are put at their eye-level.

Choose seasonal products as they are cheaper and more nutritious.

At the end of this book you'll find a template shopping list that follows the routing of most supermarkets.

Preparing Meals and Snacks

Check out the week ahead for special events when you may not have time to cook. Make extra on the days when you do have time and store the extra in the fridge or freezer so that a meal is ready when you need it. Do the same with snacks.

If you plan to go to a party or meeting, eat something before you leave home. If you go to a party or meeting on an empty stomach, you will have a very hard time resisting all the enticing food and drinks. Don't put yourself at risk for overeating and feeling guilty afterwards.

Your daily practice using the technique of prolonged pointed attention with vivid creative attention will cover after the chapter about the forth circle of healthy nutrition, "Balance", will help you with this.

The Fourth Circle of Healthy Nutrition, Balance

This section on balance again looks at food from the body's perspective. Eating good quality nutrients in moderate amounts is a crucial step toward healthy eating but doesn't necessarily cover all the needs of the body.

The circles "Quality", "Quantity" and "Timing", covered the energy-in part. In "Balance", we will cover balancing energy-in with energy-out.

Physical Activity and Basal Metabolic Rate

The energy spent on physical activity depends on our level of activity. It usually varies between 10 and 30 percent of the body's total energy expenditure but it can increase significantly beyond that at times of extreme exertion.

Basal metabolic rate, or resting metabolic rate is the energy spent to keep all the internal body systems going. This includes things like heartbeat, body temperature and digestion and takes up 70 to 90 percent of all energy used. The actual percentage depends on age, gender, bodyweight, and lean body mass and declines 2 to 3 percent per decade after the age of 35.

The function of one's metabolic system is as unique as a fingerprint. Although all metabolic systems consist of the same organs, the actual functioning differs from person to person. This explains why one

metabolic system may work at a different speed than another or why
one metabolic system may have a preference or be intolerant to certain
food items.

Going a step further, the fact that the human body is an ever-changing
organism in an ever-changing environment means that how one's
metabolic system operates from day to day and year to year depends on
the circumstances of the day and on how it ages.

How Basal Metabolic Rate Can
Lead to a Tempting Idea

Since up to 90 percent of our energy-expenditure is a result of doing
nothing else but eating and sleeping or sitting in a chair all day, it is
tempting to forget about doing regular exercise all together.

Although physical activity accounts for only a small portion of your
daily energy expenditure, continuous inactivity leads to declining
function or weakening of many body systems, which in turn leads to a
lower basal metabolic rate.

This is why regular exercise, along with healthy eating, is such an
important part of a healthy lifestyle. Both are strongly related.
Insufficient energy supply from good quality nutrients makes one feel
lethargic, missing the energy for normal daily activities and exercising.
The resulting inactivity causes one's body to deteriorate over time such
that it is no longer able to optimally metabolize the nutrients consumed.
A vicious cycle ensues.

To illustrate this important link, a 2009 issue of *"Archives of Internal
Medicine"* states:

"Four healthy lifestyle factors—never smoking, maintaining a healthy
weight, exercising regularly and following a healthy diet—together

appear to be associated with as much as an 80 percent reduction in the risk of developing the most common and deadly chronic diseases."

Three Sources of Energy to Choose from

The body generates energy required for physical activities and resting metabolic rate always from the nutrients carbohydrates, protein and fats combined in a certain ratio. This ratio changes every time the type and level of physical activity and metabolic rate change.

It is our responsibility to always provide our body with the nutrients it needs. This is accomplished by balancing the ratio of our nutrient intake with the changing demands of our body throughout a day.

The importance of maintaining this balance is the subject of the following pages. Balancing the ratio of nutrient intake is covered first with regard to the type and level of physical activity, and then with regard to metabolic rate.

Balancing the Ratio of Nutrient Intake with the Type and Level of Physical Activity

Balancing the ratio of nutrient intake with the type and level of physical activity has the objectives to avoid excessive energy intake and to preserve muscle tissue.

As mentioned above, your body always uses a combination of the macronutrients carbohydrates, fat and protein. The ratio between these nutrients changes with changes in the type and level of the physical activity.

As an example, carbohydrates are the preferred source of energy for high intensity activities, whereas fat forms the major source of energy for low intensity activities.

The table below shows which sources of energy our body prefers to tap into during various types of physical activity.

This table doesn't mention protein because, under normal conditions, protein contributes to only 1 to 2 percent of our body's energy requirement. With normal conditions, I mean the situation during which the energy requirements of the body can be easily met by the energy production of the body.

LEVEL AND TYPE OF ACTIVITY	ENERGY SOURCE
Low intensity: sleeping, reading, watching television, desk or computer work, driving a car, making yourself a lunch, stroll in the park	A combination of about 33% from carbohydrates and about 66% from fat
Ongoing moderate intensity: brisk walking, jogging, biking, canoeing	mainly carbohydrates for the first several minutes, gradually shifting after 20 to 30 minutes of ongoing activity to 50 to 60% from fat and the rest from carbohydrates
High intensity: any type of extreme exertion that causes a burning feeling in your muscles	fat and carbohydrates to the extent that the *aerobic* metabolic system can manage, and the rest from carbohydrates through the *anaerobic* metabolic system. (See below.)

Low Intensity Activities

Fat is the preferred source of energy for low intensity activities. Because both the amount of energy and the rate at which it is required are low, the body has enough time to convert fatty acids into energy. By tapping into the almost inexhaustible fat sources, the body is able to spare the more limited carbohydrate stores.

Ongoing Moderate Intensity Activities

During low to moderate intensity activities, your body uses mainly carbohydrates for the first minutes and then slowly shifts to using more fatty acids. The body emphasizes carbohydrates during the first minutes because it takes time, oxygen and extra energy to warm up the muscles and mobilize fatty acids for energy production.

While your body is mobilizing fatty acids, your body uses the carbohydrate stored in the muscle fibres. After about 20 to 30 minutes of continuous moderate intensity activity, the production of energy from fatty acids catches up with demand and enables your body to reduce the use of carbohydrates.

The amount of carbohydrate that can be stored in an average person is enough for 12 to 14 hours of rest or low intensity activity, about 2 hours of moderate intensity activity, and about 45 to 60 minutes of high intensity activities. The actual numbers depend on factors such as age and fitness level.

Being able to shift between both sources enables your body to meet its continuous energy requirements in the most economical way.

High Intensity Activities

The table shows that your body can derive 50 to 60 percent of its energy requirement from fat during moderate intensity activities. As a percentage of energy use, this is the maximum. Even though the *absolute* amount of fat metabolism may rise further when you increase your level of exertion, the amount of energy provided from carbohydrate will rise even faster.

For example,

During an hour of biking at moderate speed, you burn approximately 300 calories, about 150 from carbohydrates and 150 from fat. When you increase your cycling speed to a level where you are burning 400 calories, 240 calories or 60% come from carbohydrates and 160 calories or 40% from fat.

Your body's capability of using fat as an energy source depends on your overall condition. For an untrained person, the limit for fat mobilization is reached at 70 to 75% of maximum heart rate and, for a trained person, the limit occurs at 80 to 90% of maximum heart rate.

A simple and common used method to determine your own maximum heart rate per minute is to subtract your age from 220. For example, the maximum heart rate of someone who is 35 years old is 220 - 35 = 185. Therefore, in an untrained 35-year-old, fat metabolism has reached its maximum at a heart rate of 130 to 139 beats per minute and for a trained 35-year-old, between 148 and 166 beats per minute.

During exertion, your body is telling you that you have reached the point of deriving maximum energy from fat when your muscles begin to burn. The name for this point is lactic threshold and is the point that your body begins to activate muscle fibers connected to the *anaerobic* system to meet its energy requirement.

In part three, "Moving for Life", I go into more detail about the aerobic and anaerobic energy systems of the body and explain how they interact with muscle activity.

Putting it all Together

Knowing which energy sources the body prefers to tap into during various physical activities makes it possible to adjust food intake to achieve a match between the ratio of energy sources used and the ratio of consumed nutrients that provide that energy.

A rule of thumb for achieving that match is to eat a diet consisting of:

45 – 65% carbohydrate
10 – 35% protein
20 – 35% fat

This is a good but at the same time a rough, general guideline to use when it comes to preparing your daily meals. From here, it is all about fine-tuning the percentages to bring them in alignment with your body's requirements.

How to Balance Your Nutrient Intake during the Day

Reduce your intake of carbohydrates if you plan to perform low intensity activities. With this low level of activity, your muscles need little sugar from carbohydrates and can get most of the fuel they need from fatty acids. Therefore, focus during these conditions on protein, fat and complex carbohydrates.

Although all carbohydrates end up as sugar in your blood stream, food such as vegetables is dense and high in fiber. Consequently, they take more time to digest which slows the release of sugars into your blood stream. The carbohydrate, protein, fat ratio of your meals during these conditions should be around 1:1:1.

Try to avoid eating carbohydrates by themselves. By combining them with protein and fat, you will be slowing the speed of digestion as well as the release of sugars.

If you increase your level of activity, it is important to increase your intake of carbohydrates accordingly. Plan to have a meal about an hour and a half before working out or doing any other form of moderate or high intensity physical activity. An hour and a half works well for most people, but it can vary depending on your body's rate of digestion. Over time, you will discover what works best for you. Your meals should consist of slowly digestible complex carbohydrate, protein and fat. The ideal carbohydrate, protein, fat ratio during these conditions is around 2-3:1:1.

After an extended period of moderate to high intensity activity, it is time for recovery. If you have been working out hard, your muscles have emptied their glycogen stores and need to replenish. In addition, the body needs to repair the muscle fiber damage caused by severe physical activity.

Carbohydrates are needed to replenish the energy stores of the muscles and both carbohydrates and protein are needed to repair the muscles. Carbohydrates provide the energy and proteins provide the necessary amino acids to repair and build muscle tissue.

Your food choices after a prolonged time of physical activity depend on how hard you have been working. Focus on simple carbohydrates as in fruit combined with low-fat protein when you have been pushing yourself to the point of feeling your muscles tremble and shake. During these conditions, simple carbohydrates are a better choice since it is easier for the body to convert them into glucose than complex carbohydrates. Because fat slows down digestion, it is better to choose for low-fat protein products.

If your body doesn't get the energy from these nutrients quickly after a period of intense physical activity, it will have no choice but to break down muscle tissue into amino acids and convert these into sugar for the recovering muscles. Therefore, be sure to eat and drink within 30 minutes after completing your workout.

The carbohydrate, protein, fat ratio during these conditions should be around 2-4:1:0.

A great post-workout meal is a shake consisting of half a banana, a cup and a half green tea, a tablespoon of honey or maple syrup, and a scoop of protein powder. This has a nutritional value of about 70 grams of carbohydrates and 35 grams of protein.

Other ingredients to consider are cacao powder for anti-oxidants, magnesium and potassium, coconut oil to boost your immune system, avocados for the healthy omega-3 fatty acids and anti-oxidants, chia seeds to thicken your smoothie are a great source of protein and good fatty acids. Raw kale contains cancer-fighting ingredients and can be mixed with banana for a great taste and satiety. Goji berries are loaded with anti-oxidants. Blend them with other ingredients to take the edge off the somewhat bitter taste.

Eating low-fat food items and carbohydrates that are digested quickly must be restricted to the times of the week when you work hard. Stick to a combination of complex carbohydrates, protein and good fats at a ratio of 1 : 1 : 1 on the days you don't workout, or when your level of physical activity is only low to moderate as is the case with most endurance exercises. During these times, complex carbohydrates are metabolized fast enough to provide your body with the necessary energy.

Be careful with the amount you eat after a workout because fat cells also want to replenish themselves. You may have lost some of your body fat due to physical activity or following a low-calorie diet but the cells that *contained* the fat haven't vanished. They remain in place with the goal to recover what they have lost.

This is where many people go wrong. The feeling that they deserve a reward after completing a workout or confusing tiredness with feeling hungry combined with the strong demand of the fat cells causes many to overeat.

It requires conscious thinking, perseverance and discipline to prevent the fat cells from replenishing themselves. Use your food journal to be aware of what you eat and to prevent eating too much. Fat cells are frameworks of protein and it takes a long time before they are replaced by smaller fat cells. The body renews about 10 percent of your fat cells each year. Therefore, being successful at improving health and fitness requires a consistent, long-term healthy lifestyle.

Eating between dinner and bedtime

When your body comes to rest during the evening hours, your metabolism slows down. Although it is better not to eat before bedtime, it is hard to resist when you feel a late-night craving. Be extra careful with what you eat in the evening as it can easily undo all your hard work. A clear guideline is to avoid food that stimulates the secretion of insulin. In other words, avoid carbohydrates from other sources than vegetables or a fruit, or choose for a moderate amount of good quality, slow digesting protein that gives you the satisfied feeling you desire.

Here are some examples.

If you choose for animal based protein: chicken breast, turkey breast or light fish such as catfish, cod, trout and white tuna. Red meat is not a good choice as it induces the secretion of insulin more than white meats do.

A plant-based protein shake with lots of ice cubes.

A small piece of fruit. The fructose in fruit doesn't influence your insulin levels, burns off easily if you don't combine it with eating other food and is therefore also a good choice to get over a craving.

Vegetables are dense and high in fiber. The low insulin response combined with the slow digestion will keep you satisfied for a long time. Fruit and vegetables have the added benefit of providing vitamins, minerals, fiber and water.

Remember, limit your portion sizes, eat slowly and consciously, and know when enough is enough.

The key to a long-term healthy lifestyle is learning how to nourish your body properly from day to day during all sorts of daily activities. Choose quality food and limit your portions to provide your body with just enough fuel for your body systems to work well. Lastly, balance the ratio of nutrients with the type and level of your activity.

Keep in mind the importance of proper hydration as well.

Muscle Loss and Fat Storage are Consequences of an Imbalanced Nutrient Intake

What happens when you don't have time to eat and drink before and during high intensity activities and your carbohydrate stores run low?

In this situation, your body's only sources of energy are protein and fat. As mentioned before, it takes a lot of time and oxygen to convert fat into energy. Your body will do this as fast as it can but it will still be too slow to meet the energy demands of the muscles.

At this moment, your body begins to tap into its protein sources. Converting protein into energy is a slower process than converting carbohydrates into energy but still faster than converting fat into energy. Your body has no other choice but to literally break down muscle tissue to produce energy. This unwanted situation occurs when your body shifts into survival mode.

For our hunter and gatherer ancestors, the ability to keep fighting or running could mean the difference between life and death. What choice did they have if sacrificing body tissue for energy was their only option to stay alive? Fortunately, nowadays we hardly ever have to deal with situations of life and death that require a fight or flight reaction. However, our bodies still work in accordance with that mechanism and can't distinguish running from a bear from moving to a new house or doing a strenuous workout. After all, mechanical work is mechanical work.

Protein utilization may reach up to 15 percent of the energy production. When you take off your shirt after a long and hard workout and smell ammonia, you can draw the conclusion that at some point during your workout you emptied your glycogen stores. As a result, your body resorted to breaking down muscle tissue to produce the energy needed to continue your workout.

This is in short what happens. Protein is broken down into its smaller building blocks called amino acids and transported to the liver. The liver then removes the nitrogen molecules from the amino acids and sends the remainder back to the working muscles in the form of glucose. During this process, called deamination, the liver converts the nitrogen from the amino acid into ammonia, which then leaves the body through the kidneys or perspiration.

Again, this is an undesirable situation. You don't want to dismantle your house to feed your wood stove and you don't want to come home from a workout weaker than you were before.

The Importance of a Well-Functioning Muscular System

Muscle is a tissue worth preserving. Focus your daily activities on maintaining and building or rebuilding muscle tissue as it is the centre point of good health.

A well-functioning muscular system results in a great number of health benefits. Some examples are:

- Increased tendon and ligament strength improved joint function
- Increased bone density and improved posture, balance and stability
- Improved core strength and body control
- Improved function of the nervous system and increased metabolic rate
- Improved function of the cardiopulmonary and respiratory systems
- Reduced risk of injury during accidents and faster recovery.

Muscle - So Easy to Lose

The main factors responsible for loss of muscle tissue are aging, living a sedentary lifestyle and unbalanced eating.

The average person loses 6.6 pounds of muscle tissue every decade after the age of 35, loses 1/3 to half of his/her original muscle mass by the age of 60 and loses 12 to 14 percent of his/her strength per decade after the age of 60.

The phrase if you don't use it you'll lose it is appropriate here. Remember, your body is wired to preserve energy and is therefore not going to spend the required 30 to 50 calories per pound of muscle per day to maintain muscles you don't use and apparently don't need.

Maintaining a well-functioning muscular system can only be realized through healthy nutrition and regular exercise, the latter consisting of a combination of cardio or endurance training and strength training. The message you give your body when you exercise is that you actually need the muscles and that they therefore must be maintained.

We covered the importance of balanced eating in the chapter about the second circle of healthy nutrition, "Quantity".

Muscle, So Hard to Gain

It requires time, effort and, if you choose to go to a gym, money to keep your muscular system in good shape. The only way to build or rebuild muscle tissue is through strength training, also known as resistance training. Only overloading your muscles with resistance, in other words making them work harder than they normally do, will give your muscles the stimulus to grow in strength.

This means that activities such as walking, biking and canoeing won't help you to build or rebuild muscle tissue. Keep doing these activities if you already do them but combine them on a regular basis with strength training workouts.

In part three "Moving for Life", I go more into detail about regular exercise. Why it is important, what the relationship and difference is between strength training and cardio or endurance training and what you can do to get the best results.

Fat - So Easy to Gain

Earlier I covered what happens if you take in more carbohydrate than your muscles, brain and other body cells need or can store.

The consequence of this form of unbalanced eating is simple. Insulin will signal the liver and fat cells to pull in the glucose from the blood stream and store it as body fat. If the fat cells reach their storage capacity, insulin will simply stimulate the production of new fat cells to accommodate more fat storage.

The main factors that make gaining fat so easy are the same ones that make losing muscle tissue so easy, which are aging, living a sedentary lifestyle and unbalanced eating.

Losing 6.6 pounds of muscle tissue per decade after the age of 35 has serious consequences for your metabolic rate. As mentioned, it requires 30 to 50 calories per day to maintain a pound of muscle tissue, and these numbers will obviously increase with the increase of physical activity.

Doing the math clarifies it further, 6.6 pounds of muscle tissue times 30 calories per day equals 198 calories, which represents the number of calories you burn less every day. Not reducing your food intake accordingly makes weight gain inevitable.

With aging, your body cells, especially muscle cells, become less sensitive to insulin. This means that the ability of insulin to activate cells to pull in the glucose from the blood stream diminishes.

Fat cells never have this problem. As a result, they will have taken up most of the glucose from the blood stream before the other body cells have had the opportunity to satisfy their needs. With so many cells unsatisfied and therefore feeling hungry, you will feel hungry too with the result that you will eat more sooner than you otherwise would.

Another consequence of aging are changing hormone levels. Men produce less testosterone and women less estrogen. These hormones normally suppress the fat-storing enzymes.

Fat, So Hard to Lose

As set out earlier, when you manage to lose body fat, the cells that contained the fat are still in place.

Cells are protein structures that won't simply disappear once they lost the fat. Those structures remain where they are with the sole aim to regain what they have lost. Whenever they can, the fat cells will try to restore themselves, something at which they are very successful.

The Uniqueness of Your Metabolic System

For most people, if you let the effects of aging simply kick in without taking steps to reverse the downward spiral, it will be almost impossible to avoid weight gain and health problems.

Having said this, it is a fact that some people have a metabolic system that helps them staying lean. It seems they can eat whatever they want and never gain weight, whereas others feel that they gain weight by just looking at a piece of cake.

Fact is that being lean does not automatically equals being healthy. A lean person can have the same health problems as an overweight person such as high blood pressure, high cholesterol and diabetes. Skinny fat is the name for this health condition. Living a sedentary life style combined with unhealthy eating habits has destructive effects on every body, regardless of weight.

Regardless of the effectiveness of your metabolic system, its purpose is to ensure that nothing is wasted during the energy-in and the energy-out cycle. It is because of the body's capability to store energy efficiently and spend it economically that humankind as a species still exists.

It is through this mechanism that we have been able to withstand shorter or longer periods without food. This has been the case for over thousands of generations. Even though the world has changed and the way we live has evolved over the past 6 or 7 generations, the way our body functions remains the same.

Find Your Personal Balance

The variation among our bodies makes it impossible to come up with a one rule-fits-all solution. Factors such as age, gender, weight, genetic blueprint, type and level of physical activity and environmental circumstances require that you constantly listen to your body and do whatever is necessary to allow your metabolic system to work optimally.

Metabolic Optimum

A balanced meal contains the right ratio and amount of all the macro- and micronutrients to keep all internal systems healthy and function optimally.

There is no Metabolic System like Your Metabolic System

Since no two metabolic systems work the same, you have to understand and respect what makes your personal metabolic system thrive. In other words, you have to determine what composition of nutrients provides the best fuel and building blocks for your metabolic system.

It could be that your metabolic system prefers carbohydrate-rich food instead of protein-rich food or vice versa. The ratios among the nutrients consumed at each meal also play an important role. It all depends on your unique genetic blueprint.

The problem is that you can't examine your metabolic system. You can't see it and you can't hear it. The way to deal with this is to develop an awareness of how your body responds or talks to you. These responses can be divided into long-term and short-term responses.

Long-Term Body Responses

Examples of long-term body responses which indicate that your metabolic system is experiencing difficulty processing certain nutrients include stress, constipation, insulin resistance, weight gain, neck and back pain, poor sleep, immune system suppression, low energy, poor stamina, craving sweets, body odour, hormonal deregulation.

These examples are signals that you may have nourished your body with the wrong food. Ignoring these signals could lead to less than optimal functioning of one or more body systems, which in turn could lead to diseases ranging from something as simple as a cold to serious life threatening chronic diseases like heart diseases and cancers.

Short-Term Body Responses

Some examples of short-term body responses are nervousness, anxiety, headaches, hungry shortly after eating a meal, over-active, craving proteins or fat, difficulty concentrating, varying energy levels, feeling tired but restless, sleepy, dull, depressed mood, mentally sluggish, feeling bloated but still hungry, craving coffee and sweets.

If a meal doesn't give you energy and comfort for 3 to 4 hours, you'll need to find out which component or components of your meal were not in line with your body's metabolic requirements. The problem could be the quality, quantity, ratio of the nutrients, timing, or a combination.

You are the only true expert when it comes to finding out which nutrients in what amounts allow your metabolic system to function optimally. What may be good for another person may not be so good for you. To make it even more complicated; what works well for you today may be different next year.

The Value of a Food Log

The best way to figure out which food meets the requirements of your personal metabolic system is to keep a food log. Take the food log you used when you monitored the quantity of your food intake and add two rows per meal and snack, one for how you feel *prior* to eating a meal or snack and one row for how you feel 20 to 30 minutes *after* eating your meal or snack. Such an extended food log could look as follows:

Meal	Monday	Tuesday	Wednesday	Thursday	Friday	Saturday	Sunday
Feeling Breakfast Body Response							
Feeling Snack Body Response							
Feeling Lunch Body Response							
Feeling Snack Body Response							
Feeling Dinner Body Response							
Feeling Snack Body Response							

Every time you consume a meal or a snack, your digestive system begins to scan the food you ingest for the six nutrients. It is at this moment that you'll be able to find out which types of nutrients your digestive system prefers and which give you trouble.

Preferences or intolerances for the macronutrients carbohydrates, protein and fat can occur in endless gradations and change from year to year. Again, it is up to you to find out what your digestive system thrives on at any given stage in your life. Is it a 100 percent preference for carbohydrates and a zero percent preference for protein and fat or exactly the opposite or, most likely, something in between?

Examples of body responses after eating too many carbohydrates are nervousness, anxiety, headaches, feeling hungry shortly after eating a meal, over active, craving proteins or fat, difficulty concentrating, varying energy levels and feeling tired but restless.

Examples of body responses after eating too much protein and fat are sleepy, dull, depressed mood, mentally sluggish, feeling bloated but still hungry, craving coffee and sweets.

Body responses tell you which nutrients you should be careful with and which nutrients you should favor. After a while, you will begin to find out whether your metabolic system is a carbohydrate type, a protein-fat type or a system somewhere in between.

Nutrients, a Source of Energy or a Cause of Stress?

Eating food that leads to body responses such as those listed above are a form of stress on your body. It is important to realize that any form of stress may result in physical as well as psychological responses. As set out earlier, all aspects of health are connected to one another and imbalances in one can affect the others.

Whether stress is a result of not getting enough sleep, working too hard, moving house, divorce, the passing of a loved one, eating the wrong food or any other cause, the result is that one or more body functions will be affected to some degree.

Your body will let you know when this is the case through discomfort or pain. It is wise to address these signals before they worsen. Not by suppressing the symptoms with painkillers but by finding out what is causing the problem.

Regardless of your age or gender, your body is not supposed to hurt or be in pain. If it does, something is the matter. However, there is no need to be alarmed every time you feel something unusual. Your body is a living organism with many organs closely packed together.

Issues come and go. It is only natural. One of the major benefits of developing and training body and mind awareness is that you learn to trust your body and its ability to heal itself.

Being able to recognize and address the needs and responses of your body helps you to optimize its function and helps you to detect when something is not working optimally and is serious enough to visit a doctor. It also minimizes the chances of contracting diseases or becoming injured and in case you become ill or injured, your chances of survival will be higher and you recovery faster.

The Fifth Circle of Healthy Nutrition, Mastering Your Eating Habits

Before we dive in, let's summarize to see where we are.

In Part One we covered some basics about the nervous system, in particular the brain. How it processes the signals coming from our five senses and how the various parts of the brain play a role in the forming of beliefs, habits and expectations that ultimately shape our life.

The Two-Step technique of prolonged pointed attention with vivid creative imagination provided a method to first, replace negative thoughts to help improve our overall health and well-being and second, to consistently work on improving and strengthening our self-image.

In this we went over the four circles of healthy nutrition; "Quality", "Quantity", "Timing" and "Balance", seen from the body's perspective, meaning that we looked at the nutrients the body thrives on instead of what we would like it to thrive on.

I hope that the information so far added to your knowledge about healthy nutrition and that you feel inspired to look for ways to implement the information into your lifestyle.

The previous sentence is for many books about healthy nutrition the moment to thank you for your attention, wishing you all the best and then say goodbye.

As always, knowledge is fine and you may see the benefits of integrating that knowledge into your lifestyle, but it takes more to actually make that knowledge part of your daily behavior and life.

Going from knowing to doing, from intention to results requires a plan, a structure that will help you to go from A to B, from intention to results.

The foundation for this plan will be a solid and sound self-image. I can't emphasize enough the importance of embracing this life-long journey of self-development. It truly is a continuous process. There is always room for further improvement. It is what life is all about. It is what makes life such a beautiful experience.

The more secure and confident you feel with yourself, the easier it will be to adopt new and supportive habits that will be consistent with your goals. Developing these new and supportive habits will be the focus of the remainder of this part of the book.

Big question: what are your goals related to healthy nutrition when it comes to improving your health and quality of life?

Welcome to the process of designing a plan.

The Healthy Nutrition Plan

Here are six questions to create a well-defined outcome,

First question: is the goal specific, realistic and positive?

Be clear about what you want to achieve. "I want to lose weight" is a good start but not enough. Be specific. How much weight do you want to lose? Think of other goals such as more energy, controlling cravings, making healthy food choices.

Be sure to be realistic with regard to what you want to achieve and within what timeframe. Setting goals you hardly believe in isn't very motivating and sets you up for failure. Remember the small steps of part one.

Set a timeframe that is workable and holds you accountable at the same time. Build in time for unexpected events and delays. Things will come in your way. That's only normal, a fact of life.

Define what you *do* want, not what you *don't* want. Your subconscious mind doesn't recognize negatives and will interpret everything you think as a positive thought. As an example, when you say "I don't want to be overweight", it will focus on the word overweight and sees that as the goal to pursue.

Second question: why do I want what I want and what are the obstacles I can expect?

Does the motivation for achieving the goal come from yourself or are you stimulated by others? Your chances for success will be much bigger if the drive for realizing the desired outcome comes from within.

Do you want to achieve short-term goals such as an upcoming wedding or a vacation, or long-term goals such as maintaining an active and independent living?

Expecting that you will achieve your goals without meeting with obstacles is not realistic. In fact, obstacles are necessary for growth. Whatever their nature, they are good. "Ah, there you are" is how you welcome and embrace them. The art is to make an inventory of the obstacles you may expect to find on your path and think of strategies to deal with them. This approach will keep your mind at ease and away from stress-reactions.

Third question: when will I know that I have achieved my goal?

This may not be so difficult to answer for tangible goals such as losing 10 pounds of body fat but can be harder to answer for intangible goals such as having more energy. To answer this question you need to ask yourself what you want to feel, hear or see when you have achieved your goal.

Fourth question: what conditions are necessary to realize my goals?

Questions you need to answer: where do I go, when am I going to do it, how am I going to do it, and am I going to do it by myself or with others?

Fifth question: do I have what I need to achieve my goals?

What are the tools, skills and other recourses I now have that will help me to achieve my goals, and what more do I need?

Sixth question: is the goal I want to achieve in alignment with my intentions in life?

The deeper question you need to answer here: what is the *real* reason for my goals? How will I feel if I achieve what I want? What do I feel when I look to the future knowing that I achieved my goal? What is the best thing that could happen if I achieve my goal?

Before you can actually begin with defining your goals, you need to create a starting point. Describe where you are now with your weight, energy, unsupportive habits and so on. It is crucial to tune into reality, meaning that you have to be honest with yourself.

No need to cut corners, nobody is ever going to see what you write down if you don't want to and you accept whatever you write down without ever judging. Hold on to the Two-Step technique to allow only positive thoughts to remain kind and loving.

Spend some time on answering the questions. It is okay if you begin with a few words or short notes, you can be more elaborate any time later.

To assist you with this you'll find at the end of this book the "Lifestyle Change Goal-Setting Plan and Journal". This is a tool you can use to write down your goals following the questions above, keep track of your progress and leave comments related to challenges and successes.

Since you'll create a similar goal-setting plan for your regular workout routine in Part Three "Moving for Life", I integrated both plans in the "Lifestyle Change Goal-Setting Plan And Journal".

The goals you set in this part have a relationship with the four circles of healthy nutrition. This brings up the question about your relationship with food. What is the role food plays in your life aside of satisfying your nutritional needs?

The reason for this question is to identify emotional eating habits that may not be consistent with your health and fitness goals and therefore need to be replaced by habits that are.

Mastering Stress, Controlling Habits

Identifying the unsupportive habits you want to replace is one, implementing another. One of the first conditions needed for successfully implementing new habits is an organized day. There is no working around this. Healthy eating habits can only sustain in a week that is well structured.

The "Time-Bender" method I described on the last pages of Part One, "Mastering Your Life" helps with cleaning and organizing your days. By keeping track of all your activities during the week and reviewing your notes at the end of the week, you can pick out the activities you can delegate, re-organize, combine or terminate.

It takes a bit of time, but the pay-off is tremendous. You will find time for important activities, bring structure and rest into the days and subsequently in your mind. It creates the best conditions for cementing healthy eating habits into your lifestyle. Therefore, follow the example you'll find at the end of this book and begin.

While you are writing down your activities in segments of fifteen minutes, it may be a good idea to reflect on the habits you want to let go and on those you want to adopt.

The second habit that deserves a place on your list of good habits to install after regularly applying the "Time-Bender" method is keeping a food journal.

This is not something you need to do forever. After 4 to 6 weeks of keeping the food journal you'll have built up a good enough routine you can hold on to without writing down everything you eat and drink.

The third habit is making a weekly meal plan and having a shopping list ready at a fixed place in the kitchen. You will find both at the end of this book.

The forth habit is being aware of the short- and long-term body responses after having eaten a meal, snack or drink. The simplest way to keep track of body responses is by reserving some space on your food log.

The fifth habit is of course continuously replacing negative thoughts about yourself, others and circumstances for positive thoughts, and applying the daily practice of vivid creative imagination.

The next step is identifying the eating habits that don't support you in achieving your goals.

Negative eating habits and stress have a strong connection, which makes it obvious to look there first. Physical, mental and nutritional stress are common sources of symptoms such as those listed in the chapter "How memories, beliefs, habits and expectations take shape and cling to you".

The reason that eating and stress are so strongly connected is that food comforts and relaxes the mind and therefore works as a de-stressor. Problem is that one of the effects of stress is that the associated stress hormone cortisol desensitizes the body with the result that you need to eat more than you usual do to experience the comforting effect of eating.

This phenomenon is also part of the survival mechanism. Experiencing pain is not helpful when you need to fight or run to save your life. Even though you may have never been in such a situation or ever will be, our ancestors surely were and not feeling pain or feeling less pain could mean the difference between life or death.

Point is that the desensitizing effect of stress not only pertains to pain, but also to pleasure.

As always, awareness is the first step to change. Focus on your thoughts, feelings and behaviors and reflect whether and to what degree stress plays a role in your life. The next step will be applying the tools and skills to master these stress-reactions.

Review the symptoms and see if you can connect one or more of these symptoms with certain situations or circumstances during the day. Think of work, family, finances and relationships. Next, analyze whether these conditions affect your eating habits and if you recognize a repeating pattern. Make a list of these habits.

Trying to change stress-related habits without addressing the underlying cause isn't very effective. Using the "Time-Bender" is a first method to de-stress your life. Applying the Two-Step technique to feel good during the day and to preserve and improve a positive self-image will help you further with making the right decisions to reduce stress in your life.

Stress is a serious issue with serious physical and mental implications. Living in stress equals living in survival. I already described in Part One that one of the effects of stress is inhibiting body functions that do not play an essential part in dealing with an emergency, real or imagined, examples of which are digestion, assimilation, recovery and healing.

The second effect of stress I mentioned is that stress desensitizes the body.

Other serious effects of stress are:

- Decreased kidney function and increased salt and water retention
- Urinary loss of minerals such as calcium and boron, contributing to bone loss or osteoporosis, potassium, zinc, chromium and selenium
- Diminished number of healthy intestinal bacteria. See for the important role of intestinal bacteria Part One of this book, "How foreign invaders affect your health"
- Increased production of digestive acids in the stomach
- Deficiency in vitamins B and C
- Increased inflammatory state resulting in higher LDL or bad cholesterol, triglyceride and insulin levels

- Decreased thyroid function causing overall metabolism to slow down
- Decreased muscle mass and decreased production of the Human Growth Hormone

Looking at the health implications of stress underlines the importance of applying tools and methods to master stress responses.

Please don't try to do this through over the counter drugs, medications, binge eating, not eating at all or any other method that only deals with the symptoms but leaves the underlying cause in place.

Mastering stress in your life begins with:

- Organizing your life using the "Time-Bender" method
- Keeping a food log on which you also note body responses before and after eating and drinking
- Preparing a weekly meal plan with shopping list
- Applying the Two-Step technique consisting of step one, prolonged pointed attention to feel good every moment of the day, and step two, vivid creative imagination to improve your self-image.

These tools will help you mastering the stress reactions in your life.

More Ways to Sooth Body and Mind

The hypothalamus, part of the limbic brain controls the autonomic nervous system that further subdivides into the parasympathetic nervous system and the sympathetic nervous system. It is the latter that dominates when we are under stress and in it is the former we want to let dominate to keep body and mind relaxed and all metabolic systems run smoothly.

The reason for this quick recap is to remember that it is largely up to us to decide which of the two systems runs the show. By consciously engaging our conscious mind we have the ability to choose for actions that promote parasympathetic dominance. Fact is that when the parasympathetic nervous system dominates, stress and the associated reactions simply cannot exist.

Instead of dealing with the stress-reactions individually, we can deal with them all at once by going a step up the ladder and think of ways to influence the function of the autonomic nervous system.

Awareness is the key, setting off the continuous cycle of:

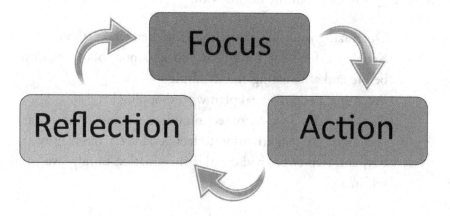

Focus-Action-Reflection

Five ways to promote parasympathetic dominance:

- Slow, deep breathing

Be aware of and observe your breathing pattern. Emotions and breathing are strongly connected. Imagine you're afraid of big black bears and you notice one close behind you when you're in a forest. Instead of slow and deep breathing from your belly, you can immediately feel your breathing go up high in your chest.

When you feel stressed, you can reduce the stress by breathing slow and deep from your belly, every exhale lasting a little longer than the inhale. By doing this you confuse your brain because it doesn't understand the breathing pattern that should be fast, high and shallow instead of slow and deep. After a while, your brain will decide to let go of feeling stressed since the signals it receives do not indicate stress.

- Recall happy and supportive thoughts and good memories

We discussed the benefits of replacing negative, stressful thoughts in Part One. It is in fact a no-brainer. Every time you are aware of negative thoughts, interrupt them. Cut them off in the middle of the sentence and replace them for happy thoughts using your safeguard. The inevitable result will be the release of feel-good neurotransmitters that result in feeling much more relaxed and at ease.

The conscious will to feel good in a world where so many people suffer is not a luxury or an act of selfishness. Nobody will ever feel any better when you feel sad or depressed. On the contrary, you will make things even worse as you will influence other people's mood.

The ongoing stream of negative thoughts and negative self-talk people allow in their mind can only lead to negative actions and habits that in turn lead to stress with all the ensuing health consequences. We have the choice to go a different path.

- Safe and effective exercising

When I mention this cure against stress, I sometimes get the question whether exercising isn't a form of stress as well. The answer is yes. The big difference is that exercising facilitates a release of physical and mental tension, which cannot take place during times you feel stressed because you're waiting in line or trying to meet a deadline.

A good workout not only depletes the stress built up during a workout but also the stress built up during the day. This makes regular exercising such a good remedy against all sorts of stress. You'll read more about safe and effective exercising in Part Three, "Moving For Life".

- Get enough sleep

We need on average eight hours of sleep per night. Getting enough hours of sleep supports many body functions that play a role in maintenance, repair, growth and detoxification, both physically as well as mentally. The pay-off is a well-rested and relaxed body that provides the best conditions for an easy operating metabolic system.

- Live clean but not too clean

Toxins can put great stress on our gut flora that to a large degree determine our health, both physically and mentally. Although it is almost impossible to avoid all toxins, we can minimize their impact on our health by choosing for products that carry the least amount of chemicals.

This pertains to food and drinks and to everything in our environment ranging from air and water to clothing, cosmetics, carpets and furniture. All sorts of influences can set off stress-reactions in the body.

On the other hand, living too clean can have its drawbacks as well. The cleaner we live due to our dietary choices, use of antibiotics, anti-bacterial soaps and disinfectants the less diverse and therefore the less healthy our microbiome will be. Since the latter plays an important role in regulating the immune response, the consequence of a compromised microbiome will be a compromised immune function with all possible ensuing physical and mental consequences.

Avoid toxins but don't be too afraid for a bit of dirt on your hands when you are outside working in your garden for instance. We have evolved with a wide variety of bacteria on and in our body and we need them to keep our immune system balanced and free from stress.

Five strategies that suppress the sympathetic and promote the parasympathetic nervous system you can add to your list of supporting habits.

As I mentioned before, I don't know your life situation. I don't know where you have gone through and where you are now. Therefore, if these five recommendations can't help you with reducing stress to a level you can master, look for additional tools and people whose daily work it is to help people with mental issues and follow their recommendations.

Making Supportive Eating Habits Part of Your Healthy Life Style

Summarizing the supportive habits you can put on your list of habits to make part of your healthy lifestyle:

- Organizing your life using the "Time-Bender" method
- Keeping a food log on which you also note body responses before and after eating and drinking
- Preparing a weekly meal plan with shopping list
- Slow, deep breathing from your belly
- Recalling happy and supportive thoughts and good memories using the 24/7 safeguard technique of prolonged pointed attention
- Safe and effective exercising, see Part Three of this book
- Getting enough rest and sleep
- Avoid toxins but don't live too clean

Make a second list of habits you want to replace because they are holding you back from achieving your goals.

The following step is creating a strategy to implement the supportive and replace the negative habits.

Prioritizing is key. It is will not work to address them all at the same time. Begin with the first three habits of the list of supportive habits and add one habit from your list of negative eating habits you want to replace.

For example, if you want to wean off from eating unhealthy food and drinks, choose consciously for implementing the habit of eating healthy food and drinks.

Use the Two-Step technique to cement healthy eating habits into your lifestyle. Remember to do it gradually, in other words take small steps.

The first step is consciously thinking throughout the day for a few days about the habits you want to install and/or replace. You have become familiar with the Step-One safeguard technique prolonged pointed attention to fill your mind with positive thoughts, and now you want to use this same Step-One technique to become familiar with the nature of the new habits.

It is all about preparing yourself. Give it a few days if you need to. Think about how these new habits and of their positive effect on all aspects of your life. As always, keep a positive mind. See it as part of the process, so enjoy it.

Think of the runway and flight plan I mentioned in the preface. It really doesn't make any sense to tell you to just do it, even though it may sound logic. Humans aren't always logic and life isn't always logic.

About the last place where you can expect logic is in the subconscious mind, housing in the limbic system, the hot area of the brain where emotions rule. Your subconscious mind is not the area you can enter with your conscious mind in the role of a traffic police officer, expecting everybody and everything to obey quickly to your clear commands.

Expect a big riot instead with the subconscious mind as the eventual winner.

You may expect better results when you play the emotional card here. Think of an approach including acceptance, compassion, optimism, encouragement, flexibility, gentle persistence and patience.

Welcome to step two, applying the technique of vivid creative imagination.

Picture again that big white screen in front of you and project yourself onto the screen going through a normal day before implementing any of the new habits. Let this picture then disappear to the right, representing the past, and move in from the left side of the screen, representing the present, a picture of you performing the new habits as if they already are part of your everyday life.

Do this as vividly and as detailed as possible to promote the release of the feel-good neurotransmitters, your big allies that support you in the process. To enhance the experience, go into the screen and into yourself and look out of your eyes while you are performing these tasks and habits.

Use your senses. Look very carefully at all the details. See yourself sitting at the table reviewing the Time-Bender, and preparing your weekly meal plan and shopping list. Know which day it is as well as the moment of the day. Can you hear music in the background and do you have coffee or tea in front of you on the table? Put it all and more there.

See through your eyes when you're doing errands, and make your healthy food choices. Put in the details of the environment. See and feel the healthy products you will buy, think of the meals they will be part of, how much you will enjoy these meals and how grateful your body and mind will be. Still walking through the supermarket, be aware of what you hear, feel, smell and see.

Back home see how, when and where you prepare a meal. Look, feel, smell, hear and taste. Consciously engage all your five senses. When you eat your meal, be aware of the positive comments you give yourself and hear from others. Fill in the entire environment using your senses.

After finishing your meal, notice how well you nourished your body and mind. Think further than the act of eating alone and think the entire experience, which includes the environment, how nice warm it was, the people you were with the pleasant conversations and so on.

Make the entire experience as real and vivid as you can and as if it is already a reality. It is essential to keep this in mind as it will help to ingrain the associated habits as quickly as possible. Don't hold back and get excited for that will induce the neurotransmitters that will help you with this process.

When you're finished with that days' practice, go back to Step One to hold on to the good feelings and intentions for the rest of the day, act upon them and create an ongoing cycle of Step One and Step Two, day after day.

Similar to Part One, using affirmations is another way to reach your brain in order to install or replace supportive habits. The affirmation below consists again of three parts. The function of the second and third part is to reinforce the previous part.

"I feel confident, happy and safe because I see myself on my way to installing healthy eating and life style habits. I can feel that my body and mind are healthier, stronger and more energetic because of the healthy food I eat and drink. I am organizing my days using the Time-Bender, fill out my food journal every day, prepare a meal plan every week and have a shopping list at a fixed place in the kitchen to make my shopping more efficient. I notice that by structuring my days, I feel relaxed and in control of my actions and habits. I know with certainty that these new habits make me look and feel healthy and happy every day and make me perform at my best every day. I will hold on to these new habits because that is what I want to do for the rest of my life."

"Because, I remember every moment of the day to plan and organe my days, I realize how much more relaxed, confident and in control of my days, habit and lifestyle choices I am. I am enjoying my meals, focus on and listen to my body's responses and make adjustments in my food choices to feed my body even better because I know that my body will reward me with feeling and looking better every new day. I am aware of the positive effects of healthy eating and lifestyle habits and how they empower me to keep me on track toward achieving and maintaining a rewarding and fulfilling healthy, active and independent happy life."

"I feel better every day and fully enjoy creating the life I choose to live."

Use the Step-Two vivid creative imagination practice and the affirmations as concepts to adjust to your own situation. The variations can of course be endless.

A few rules to keep in mind:

Stay in the present, as if the desired outcome is already a fact. To give an example: do not say things like "I'm going to" or "Next time I will". Words like these point toward a desired outcome in the future.

Avoid negatives because they unconsciously set you up for failure and frustration. Examples are cannot, try, could have, but, might, should, would have, must, maybe, couldn't, some day.

Record the script and listen to it three to four times. Although you may find listening to your own voice a bit awkward, don't let these emotions get between you and your goals. The pay-off is two-fold. First, your brain can concentrate on one action which is listening and second, the fact that you are listening to your own voice makes the affirmation much more effective.

Focus, Action, Reflection and Repeat

Some things to consider before moving on the final part of this book.

Healthy eating and drinking can be achieved only by working on all the circles of health consistently and simultaneously. Leave one out and you are likely to go off track fast. Compare it to driving your car. Unless you pay attention to holding the steering wheel, other traffic, road signs, and weather conditions all at the same time, you are not likely to reach your destination.

Your body is not a machine and won't always agree with what you think or want it to do. Losing weight and improving health does not happen overnight and it is not a linear process. You may plan to lose one or two pounds every week but your body goes by its own schedule. It may go faster or slower than you had planned and it may even come to a standstill or go backwards. So be it. Accept it, be patient, hold on to what you know is good and have fun with the process.

Everybody hits plateaus when it seems impossible to get the body moving again. Simply sit down and figure out what is going on. Ask yourself:

-   Do I really eat and drink good quality food?

You may allow yourself to indulge in convenience food now and then when you are young, but not when you are in your forties and you have reached the phase in your life that your metabolism slows down and your strength and activity levels decline.

-   Do I really limit my portion sizes sufficiently?

No matter how healthy you eat, you will gain weight if you eat more than your body needs. Even though you may feel 100 percent convinced that you don't eat too much, the fact that you're not losing weight may indicate the opposite. Remember that you have to respect and follow your body's pace. Hold on to the technique described in step one of feeling good and preparing yourself for implementing new habits, replacing unwanted habits and adjusting existing habits.

-   Do I time my eating and drinking correctly?

Your body requires good quality food and fluids starting with a good breakfast. Anything less will challenge the smooth function of your metabolic system. Preparing weekly meal plans will surely help you with this.

-   Do I balance my food intake correctly with the type and level of my physical activities and my metabolic optimum?

Eating food that your body can't digest well or that is not in line with the type and level of your physical activity may cause your metabolism to become imbalanced. The effects on the body can be both physical and mental, ranging from weight gain to muscle loss to a decrease in energy, mood swings, and cravings.

-   Do I really focus on my goals and am I listening well to the needs of my body?

Consciously or unconsciously, people are lead astray by a myriad of factors. Consistently using the Two-Step meditation technique and maintaining the ongoing routine of Focus – Action – Reflection will help you to stay on track.

At the end of this book you will find a checklist for achieving and maintaining a healthy weight. This checklist goes by all the five individual circles and their important topics and helps you to determine whether there is room for improvement on any of them.

How to Stay Motivated. Hold on to your Anchors

When everything is going your way, you rarely need support or motivation. Prepare yourself for the times when you may struggle.

The moment you find yourself in the midst of such a struggle, hold on to the anchors we already discussed:

- Time-Bender
- Food and Fluid Journal
- The Weekly Meal Plan + Shopping List
- Template Shopping List
- Checklist Achieving and Maintaining a Healthy Weight
- The Two-Step technique of Prolonged Pointed Attention combined with Vivid Creative Imagination
- The affirmations

Three more anchors that will help you stay on track:

- A Lifestyle Change Goal-Setting Plan and Journal

I already mentioned this plan and journal in which you write about the changes you have already implemented and the ones you are planning to make. You can use a notebook for this journal or the template you will find at the end of this book. It is a great tool for keeping track of your overall progress as it will keep you focused on your goals and help you to cement your new habits into your lifestyle.

- A support system

Another excellent method to stay motivated and committed is going public with your goals. Social support puts positive pressure on you to keep yourself on track.

Tell your family and friends about your journey and that you expect them to support you. Keep them updated on your successes and challenges. A good support system will help you achieving your goals faster than trying to do it all on your own.

And why not take it up a level? Find someone who also wants to improve her or his health and work for a strong and lean body. Hold each other accountable, work out together, plan your meals together, and keep each other motivated and on track.

- A reward system

Reward yourself for successes. Not with food of course but with new clothes, a book or beginning an activity that contributes to your self-development such as learning to play a musical instrument or any other hobby.

Whenever it gets hard to keep yourself going, think about the reason you originally wanted to get back in shape. Was it for yourself, was it to be a good example for your kids or your grandchildren, was it for your husband, your wife, your friends?

Think of those reasons and write them down, again and again if that helps.

Some Final Thoughts

For anything to work in this book it is imperative to maintain an undercurrent of kindness. In other words, remain in a state of relaxation no matter what. As soon as you allow any form of stress in your life because you feel disappointed, frustrated or even angry at yourself or others, you are always and instantaneously moving yourself away from your health goals.

Be aware of where you are throughout the day. Catch yourself. What are you thinking? Where are you now? What are you doing? Is this what I want to do? Is this where I want to be? And so on. Apply the routine of

Focus – Action – Reflection and use the Safeguard technique to replace negative thoughts and feelings.

Rely on your conscious mind for that is your only key to change. Your conscious mind can only work in the present. The past is the past and can't be undone. Look at your experiences as feedback and opportunities to learn from and then forget about them. There is no future in digging in the past.

Through using your conscious mind you can create the circumstances for a better future. Accept an unwanted situation you find yourself in and make conscious decisions on the best steps to take. This excludes questions sounding like "why don't things go the way I want?" "Why is this happening to me?" "Why always me?"

Questions like these drive you straight into stress-mode with the risk that you will lose yourself in some kind of petty party that will only lead you away from where you want to be.

Instead of "why?", ask yourself "what?". "What can I do to improve the situation I'm in?" This question makes you grab the conductor's stick and puts you in charge.

Accepting a situation as it is keeps your mind relaxed and helps your conscious mind with clear thinking and making the right decisions. This is the moment where willpower enters the picture. Willpower is the conscious mind's crown jewel and a great feature to pursue our goals, but only if applied wisely.

Willpower is often connected to pushing through no matter what. Even though this strategy may work in the short term, it will never work in the long term. Using an example may explain best why.

Suppose I politely ask someone to step aside so that I can pass. If the other person is not willing, he will simply reply with "no". Suppose I persist and repeat the question with more force in my voice. If the other person is still not willing to move out of the way, he will reply with a force at least as forceful as mine. This can continue going back and forth to a point that I begin pushing or pulling to get him out of the way. What will he do if he is still not willing to do cooperate? Dig in his heels, hold on to something, sit down on the floor?

You get the picture. In this example, I played the role of the conscious mind and my opponent that of the subconscious mind.

The take away, don't change or fight a negative habit by using a strategy of attack, suppression, aggression, punishment or any type of tension. You might as well better stop right away for you're wasting your time and energy and will eventually fail anyway.

Using willpower negatively will only draw extra attention to the negative habit and therefore make it stronger.

Through using the intelligence of your conscious mind wisely, you can master your willpower and use it effectively. Instead of acting like the traffic police officer I mentioned before, understand that the subconscious mind is all about emotions and much stronger than your conscious mind. Gentle persistence forms the core of your strategy to get what you want.

Making sound choices and persisting gently are actions of your conscious mind using willpower positively and wisely.

When applied the right way, the conscious mind doesn't give in or up but focusses on and reflects upon the situation from a relaxed and intelligent perspective. It accepts the negative habit for the moment but remains focused and persistent in finding strategies to replace the habit.

Not by trying to eradicate or overpower the negative habit but by remodelling the habit. Think of rewarding yourself with a healthy snack instead of a sugary treat or with something other than food.

Positive willpower uses the 10 anchors mentioned above. Honor and use your conscious mind to master and use your willpower wisely. Work with focus to kindly, lovingly, patiently, persistently and consistently install positive habits, one by one and one step at the time.

Remind yourself that the forming of new neural pathways is a physical process that you don't need to question. It works. Trust it, surrender to it, create the circumstances, let it happen and create your victory.

Part Three

"Moving For Life"

"Exercise is King, nutrition is Queen, put them together and you've got a kingdom."

Jack LaLanne

Introduction and Overview

Building a healthy physique is takes time and dedication and is therefore, similar to what I wrote about healthy nutrition, nothing less than a journey of learning and experiencing. The method to building a healthy, energetic and strong physique with all body organ systems working at their best, is through forms of physical activity that are safe, effective, efficient and enjoyable.

But regardless of the form, physical activity alone is not enough to build a healthy body as this can only occur if it is provided with the right nutrients at the right time. This makes healthy nutrition an indispensable partner of physical activity.

Similar to healthy nutrition, safe and effective exercising also consists of five circles. It begins with explaining the relationship between health and fitness, and goes into the four elements of fitness that play a role in achieving and maintaining good health.

The follow-up covers the muscular system, the first and most important element of fitness and center point of good health. The unique quality of the muscular system lies in its ability to pull *all* other body systems forward in their function. This effect depends entirely on the state of the muscular system and works therefore in two ways. Whether its function improves or declines, *all* other body functions will follow suit.

Stimulating the muscular system in a way that it gradually grows in strength and size requires specific forms of physical activity. After considering the positive effects of a well-maintained muscular system, we'll cover the laws and principles that need to be respected in order to ensure safe, effective, efficient and enjoyable training.

The next step will be creating a plan that represents the core of working toward achieving and maintaining a healthy, strong and energetic body. You will read about a six-step effective exercise plan, following the same format as used in the previous part about healthy nutrition. It will serve as your roadmap to arrive safely at the point of destination.

With all the preparations taken care of, it is time for action. "Moving for Life" offers you a full body workout with variations. It also gives clear descriptions of the exercises with accompanying pictures to perform the exercises correctly.

The function of the fifth circle "Mastering Your Exercise Habits" is similar to the fifth circle in "Eating for Life" in the sense that it offers you essential tools to keep you focused and on track toward your personal health and fitness goals with a regular workout routine.

The guide ends with combining all three parts of this book into a solid partnership, your foundation for achieving and maintaining good health for the rest of your life.

Read the entire guide first to become familiar with the content and then go back to the chapter explaining your personal six-step effective exercise plan.

The Five Circles For Save and Effective Exercising

The Fundamental Laws of Strength Training The fundamental laws form the core of healthy exercising. It refers to the big rocks that together form the foundation of every strength training program.

The Principles of Strength Training The principles of strength training build further upon the fundamental laws. Following the principles mentioned in this section supports a gradual and continuous improvement of overall strength.

The Six-Step Effective Exercise Plan A plan is like a roadmap you rely on when you travel from one place to another. Starting a journey without proper planning is nothing less than preparing for failure. This third circle covers the six simple but important steps to ensure that you have a sound plan in place before moving to the next phase.

The Full Body Workout The next phase is the fourth circle and goes into the physical preparation and the ins and outs of the workouts and your training program. This is where all the real action happens. Planning is essential, but planning without action is only daydreaming. Implementing the components of the six-step effective exercise plan and following through is what eventually produces the results you're after, nothing else.

Mastering Your Exercise Habits The fifth and last circle completes the picture. Unless we teach our mind to do what is good for the body we remain trapped in a detrimental lifestyle. The aim is to bring balance to body and mind in a way that they support one another.

Balance among all six aspects of health is not something that can be achieved and maintained with short-term goals and actions. Health lasts a life time and is therefore a long-term endeavor. Only by consistently being aware of what your body needs throughout the stages of your life and acting accordingly can you maximize your potential to live a long and healthy independent life. The only appropriate strategy for this is to implement a lifestyle that suits all aspects of your personal wellness wheel.

Health and Fitness

Health and fitness are often named in one and the same breath and with good reason for they are strongly related. But being strongly related is something else than being the same.

Both terms are defined in many ways. If you search the internet you'll find many different interpretations.

Health is often defined as metabolic efficiency or not having a disease or sickness. Health is a wide concept and comprises more than only physical health. Think of the mental and emotional, social, relationships, spiritual, professional and financial aspects I mentioned in "Eating for Life".

Health

For thousands of years, health has always been the first condition for humankind to survive as a species and to pass on DNA to the next generation. The absence of health almost certainly meant an early death, leaving only those in good health the chance to produce offspring. This simple harsh rule of Mother Nature is the reason humankind could successfully compete with other species, withstand environmental conditions and secured its existence.

This function of health never changed even though we don't have to fear an early death when we lack good health. We also don't have to fight against lions, bears and extreme weather conditions anymore. What has changed is how we perceive health. Nowadays, health stands for being able to live a long, happy, active and independent life.

Fitness

Fitness can be defined as being able to perform physical activity.

In other words, the higher our level of fitness, the better our condition, the more we can physically handle. It is obvious that zero level fitness equals death.

The function of fitness is to serve health, our greatest personal treasure. This forms the foundation of the relationship between health and fitness. Both should go hand in hand but can easily grow apart.

You negatively affect your health when you increase your level of fitness to a degree where your body is no longer capable of recovering from ongoing exertions.

Examples are the sportsmen and women who push their body to the limit, and sometimes beyond. They build their whole life around their sport and do everything to improve their performances. By putting such a strain on their body, they constantly run the risk of becoming injured. The injury can be acute as with spraining an ankle or occur more gradually in the form of overuse.

On the other hand, you also affect your health in negatively when you let your level of fitness *drop below* the point where your bodily functions cannot longer work properly. Physical inactivity and wrong eating habits are more often than not responsible for this situation.

In this case, sudden exertions such as with running to catch a bus, climbing stairs, an upsetting phone call or snow shoveling can get someone's health in serious trouble, which is exactly the situation too many people are dealing with in today's society.

Fitness must be at a level where your health benefits most as it offers the best quality of life possible. Good for you and your loved ones, now and in the long run.

The Four Elements of Fitness

The four elements of fitness are the cardiorespiratory system, the muscular system, flexibility and body composition.

The Cardiorespiratory System

The cardiorespiratory system consists of the cardiovascular system, heart, arteries and veins, and the respiratory system, from mouth and nose to the lungs.

The respiratory system adds oxygen to the blood and removes carbon dioxide from the blood. At the same time, the cardiovascular or circulatory system transports the oxygen together with nutrients and hormones to the body tissues and removes waste.

Both systems work in close harmony. About 5 litres of blood circulate in an adult every minute when at rest, to 6 or 7 times a minute during maximal exercise. The rate of respiration is approximately 10 litres of air per minute when at rest to 60 litres during exercise. Well-trained athletes use over 200 litres per minute. The air we breathe contains about 21 percent oxygen. The actual oxygen uptake depends on factors such as gender, body mass and overall condition. To give an indication, the oxygen uptake during exercise of an aerobically fit male weighing 70 kg is about 4 litres per minute and for an unfit male weighing the same about 2.5 litres per minute.

The respiratory system is a complex and amazingly efficient system that works 24 hours a day year after year to keep us alive and to let us do the things we want to do.

Obviously, the stronger the cardiorespiratory system, the better it works, the longer it lives. Like any system, it requires good maintenance. If not, it deteriorates and breaks down.

The only method to keep the cardiorespiratory system in good condition is through a combination of proper exercising and healthy nutrition.

Some benefits of a cardiorespiratory system in good shape:

- Increased amount of blood ejected from the left ventricle of the heart with every beat. The effect is an increased delivery of oxygen and nutrients to the body tissues and a lower resting heart rate.
- Increased number of red blood cells which transport oxygen carrying hemoglobin to the body tissues.
- Increased density of capillaries, the smallest and most numerous of blood vessels. An increased density means a better distribution of oxygen and nutrients and an improved waste removal.
- Increased size and number of mitochondria. Mitochondria, called the powerhouses of the cell, are little organelles in a cell that use oxygen and are responsible for the production of energy created from the food and fluid we consume.
- Increased aerobic enzymes resulting in an enhanced ability to utilize oxygen.

When reading these points, it makes sense that insufficient cardiorespiratory training leads to the opposite results. A body with a poor cardiorespiratory condition is in trouble when it meets with a challenge it can't withstand. Taking a rest is one method to prevent the system from breaking down, avoiding challenges altogether another.

But what if the challenge comes unexpectedly or can't be controlled as is the case with accidents, periods of extreme cold or hot weather, illnesses or fierce emotions? It is not difficult to think of more examples that are part of normal daily living, nor is it hard to imagine what the consequences under these circumstances will be for a cardiorespiratory system out of shape.

Having your cardiorespiratory system in good condition is extremely important to be able to withstand challenges, to feel healthier and to have a better quality of life.

The Muscular System

The human body consists of more than 600 muscles, attached to bones by tendons. The muscular system makes us capable to perform a variety of actions by contracting and becoming shorter. That is all muscles can do. They pull but they can't push.

Skeletal muscle is the most abundant tissue in the body, making up about 23 percent of a woman's body weight and about 40 percent of a man's body weight.

Each muscle gets its instructions from the nervous system that is composed of the central nervous system (CNS) and the peripheral nervous system (PNS). Another function of the latter is to continuously deliver information about all body parts to the CNS, the brain and the spinal cord, for processing.

The interaction between the muscular system and the nervous system makes out how we move and is subject to the study called kinesiology, the science of anatomy in action.

Because the only thing muscles can do is contracting means that they need opposing muscles to bring them back in resting length.

For example, when the bicep muscles at the front side of the upper arm contract, they need the triceps muscles at the backside of the upper arm to oppose that movement. This makes the biceps the prime mover or the agonist and the triceps the antagonist. A third category, the synergists are the stabilizing muscles that need to contract to reduce or prevent undesirable movements that may occur while the agonist and the antagonist are at work. An example of stabilizing muscles are the core muscles that need to contract in order to give the body stability when doing for instance biceps curl exercises.

It is important to realize that all muscles can play the role of agonist, antagonist or synergist. It just depends on the specific movement.

In relation to fitness, it makes sense that the better one's muscular capacity, the more it contributes to one's level of fitness. Muscular capacity comprises strength, endurance, speed, coordination and flexibility and give combined the following results:

Strength and Endurance	=	Muscular Endurance
Speed and Endurance	=	Speed Endurance
Strength and Speed	=	Power

Agility and mobility combine coordination, flexibility and power.

Muscles contribute to the level of fitness in more ways than with just movement, strength, endurance and power. Muscles are the real motor of human body in the sense that the better their condition, the better the condition of the human body as a whole.

If muscles get stronger, the other body systems cannot stay behind, they must follow accordingly. If, through training, you would only improve your muscular system, you would likely tear your body apart on the first forceful contraction of your muscles if not also your bones, tendons and ligaments had not become stronger as well. In other words, a well-developed muscular system leads to:

- increased bone, tendon and ligament strength
- improved joint function or flexibility
- increased bone density, helping to prevent osteoporosis
- improved balance and stability
- improved core strength, included reduced low-back pain and posture
- improved body control and awareness
- improved function of the nervous system
- Increased metabolic rate
- increased cardiovascular and cardiorespiratory condition
- reduced body fat
- reduced risk of injuries and faster healing and recovery

These are just some of the benefits. Since all bodily systems are connected, all will develop and improve proportionally with the improvement of the muscular system. Realize however that the opposite is also true; a weak muscular system leads to weak body systems.

Flexibility

Flexibility is a measure of the range of motion around a joint, for example the elbow, or a number of joints, like the lower back. The range of motion is limited by the physical structure of the joint including the bones, tendons, ligaments and muscles.

Flexibility is essential when performing everyday activities and therefore an important component of fitness.

Three categories of joints:

- Fibrous joints are joints that don't allowing any movement. Think of the bones of the skull or pelvis.
- Cartilaginous joints are attached to each other by cartilage. These joints allow little movement, such as in the spine and ribcage
- Synovial joints are joints that are the freely movable and the most commonly known joints

Synovial joints have cartilage along the surface of the bones to reduce friction and to absorb shocks. They are enclosed by a capsule that holds a lubricating fluid.

The three major types of synovial joints are:

- Hinge joints, which allow movement in one direction, like the elbow and the knee joints
- Condyloid joints, which move in two directions, like wrist and ankle joints
- Ball and socket joints move in three directions and have the largest range of motion. Examples are the shoulder and hip joints

Flexibility training is a controversial topic among athletes and their trainers. Some promote it and some reject it. Both camps have their experts.

Most experts agree that it is not wise to perform static stretches prior to a workout when muscles, ligaments and tendons are not yet warm and pliable. If you do, you are asking for trouble. It is better and even essential to warm-up the body before stretching or a workout with dynamic movements that gradually build up in intensity.

It is to this point that the majority of the experts agree.

When it comes to flexibility training after a workout two main visions prevail.

Those who support flexibility training after a workout say stretching:

- Reduces stress in the muscles and releases tension developed during the workout
- Assists with posture by balancing muscle tension across joints
- Reduces the risk of injury during training and daily activities
- Improves the performance during training and daily activities

The opponents value flexibility as much as those who support it but argue that flexibility training should be part of proper exercising.

When you stretch, you apply force on a muscle at the farthest end of its range of motion. Exercising properly means you are moving the joints through their full range of motion, and achieve the same results as with stretching after a workout.

Flexibility is different for everybody. It is mainly a matter of genetics and similar to one's ability to run or bike faster than others. Being different is no problem, it is only normal.

Problems with flexibility are in most cases a symptom of a muscular system that is under performing. Proper exercising enhances joint function and brings one's joints, bones, ligaments and tendons, in the best possible condition.

If you want to stretch after a workout because you feel it benefits you, then do so but stay within the same range of motion as during the resistance exercises. Let it never be painful, breathe normally and don't try to do things with your joints your body is not capable of.

Body Composition

Body composition is the proportion of fat free mass to fat mass.

Fat free mass is muscle, bone, blood, organs, and fluid.

Fat mass is adipose or fat tissue located under the skin and around organs.

The two elements of body composition we all focus on are fat and muscle. Losing body fat and gaining muscle is the common goal for most people who want to improve their fitness.

People with too much body fat have a higher risk of heart disease, high cholesterol, high blood pressure, stroke, diabetes, digestive and pulmonary disorders, joint problems and so on.

Too much body fat means that the body has to work harder to keep all systems functioning. Overexerting the body leads to extra wear and tear, increasing the risk of a breakdown in one or more body systems leading to health issues ranging from acute injuries to chronic diseases.

Research learned that it is not so much the total amount of fat that determines the risk for developing health issues, but more where the fat is located in the body. Visceral fat, the fat in the trunk area around organs, is of greater risk than evenly distributed fat under the skin.

Visceral fat produces and releases 24/7 inflammatory signals into the blood stream, leading to heart disease, stroke, colon cancer, dementia, hypertension, diabetes and rheumatoid arthritis.

Men and women with belly fat are also more likely to have more plaque in their arteries, insulin resistance, type-2 diabetes and abnormal cholesterol levels.

Belly fat also produces the female hormone estrogen in both men and women, which adds to the risk of breast cancer for women and stimulates the forming of breast tissue in males, known as men boobs.

Determining one's health risk by only measuring one's total percentage of body fat, which is a commonly used method, is therefore not very useful. It doesn't say where the fat is located. Other methods of measuring body fat have drawbacks as well.

Skinfold measurements measure the thickness of a double fold of skin and underlying fat, but don't measure internal fat.

Girth measurements measure the total circumference of either limbs or the trunk but include skin, fat, muscle and bone all at the same time.

A body mass index (BMI) only measures the ratio between body weight and body length at a predetermined level based on averages. But what if someone has more muscles than average because of regular strength training?

Combining several types of measurements done on a regular basis is the best method to estimate one's health risk. If, for instance, skinfold measurement goes down and girth goes up, then the muscle has grown. If both skinfold and girth goes up, then girth has grown because of increased fat and *possibly* of increased muscle. Another very helpful and fast tool to determine whether you carry too much body fat is being honest to yourself while standing naked I front of a mirror.

Improving the Muscular System

The only way to improve the function of the four elements of fitness is through muscle activity and healthy nutrition, which explains the important role of regular physical activity and supportive eating habits. A sedentary life style, often accompanied by unhealthy eating habits, directly affects one's fitness level and subsequently one's health.

This chapter is about the different types of muscle fiber, their function and the type of exercises that help to improve and maintain their function and in turn overall health.

Muscle Fibers, Slow Twitch and Fast Twitch

A big misconception is that we have and use one type of muscle for the various activities of daily life. Truth of the matter is that muscle tissue consists of two main groups of muscle fiber types:

Type 1 muscle fibers, also known as slow twitch or endurance muscle fibers, and type 2 muscle fibers, also known as fast twitch or strength muscle fibers.

Both muscle fiber types are connected to specific physical activities. Comparing both muscle fiber types in the diagram below shows how much they differ from each other.

Strength/Type 2/Fast Twitch Muscle Fibers	Endurance/Type 1/Slow Twitch Muscle Fibers
Poor in endurance, high in strength.	High endurance, poor in strength
Develop short, forceful contractions	Develop long, continuous contractions
Speed and power	Endurance
Only recruited by the central nervous system during high-intensity work	Recruited by the central nervous system during low-intensity work
Recover slow	Recover fast
Work without the use of oxygen (anaerobically)	Work with the use of oxygen (aerobically)
White color due to the absence of oxygen carrying red blood cells	Red color due to the presence of an abundance of oxygen carrying red blood cells

We need the fast twitch muscle fibers for strength and for times we need to fight or flight. This means translated to modern daily circumstances that we need fast twitch muscle fibers for activities such as carrying our shopping bags, maintaining good posture and walking stairs, and the fight and flight ability of these muscle fibers to catch a bus or to keep ourselves on our feet when we trip.

The slow twitch muscle fibers are important for ongoing low to moderate intensity activities ranging from sleeping and sitting to walking the dog and vacuuming.

Males and females have identical muscular systems. Both are equipped with about 50 percent slow twitch and 50 percent fast twitch muscle fibers. The fiber type distribution is also the same. It's one's gender, age, genetic blueprint and type and level of physical activity that largely accounts for the size and strength of the fibers.

Preserving energy is an important reason for the existence of these two muscle fiber types. Slow twitch muscle fibers consume less energy than fast twitch muscle fibers. The central nervous system, the system that controls voluntary muscle contractions therefore always activates slow twitch muscle fibers first.

The CNS only activates the energy-expensive fast twitch muscle fibers when we need to overcome a resistance that exceeds 25 percent of our maximum strength.

This effect is called the size principle, meaning that muscle fibers are recruited from smallest to largest, always beginning with the slow twitch muscle fibers.

This is what it looks like in a table where the rectangle represents the total of muscle fibers in a body:

Strength   **Muscle Fibers**

75%	About 50% **FAST TWITCH** muscle fibers Strength / type 2 / Anaerobic, glycolytic / White High in strength Activated when using 25% - 100% of maximum strength Big in size, slow recovery
25%	About 50% **SLOW TWITCH** muscle fibers Endurance / type 1 / Aerobic, oxidative / Red High in endurance Activated when using less than 25% of maximum strength Small in size, quick recovery

The fact that the CNS only activates the fast twitch muscle fibers when we need more than 25 percent of our maximum strength means that these fast twitch muscle fibers remain dormant when the level of physical activity stays below the 25 percent threshold. They even won't take over the task from the endurance muscle fibres when the latter get tired.

If You don't Use It, You'll Lose it....

Another principle enters the picture at this moment: if you don't use it you'll lose it. Because muscle tissue is metabolic active tissue, meaning that the body has to spend energy to maintain muscle tissue, strength or fast twitch muscle fibers that aren't used on a regular basis will be broken down.

Spending energy on maintaining muscle fibers you don't use equals wasting energy and is not in line with how the body is wired. The response of the body is that it begins to break down what is causing the waste of energy. In other words, it begins to break down precious muscle tissue.

This natural process already automatically occurs when we age. When we reach the age of 35, we hit the phase in life called somatopause. From this point in life on our body begins to break down muscle tissue, a result of declining human growth hormone (HGH) levels. The muscle tissue that wastes away amounts on average 6.6 pounds per decade. This process speeds up the older we get and men lose more than women. By the age of 60, about a third to half of the original muscle tissue may have disappeared. Think of the men and women that live in retirement homes to realize the effect of muscle tissue breakdown.

This effect was never a real problem for our ancestors since they never got older than 40 or 50. Life expectancy nowadays is much longer, which is a true privilege but a privilege that comes with the responsibility to keep our body in good condition. Maintaining our HGH levels becomes increasingly important when we age to prevent our body from deteriorating disproportionally fast. The direct result if we don't will be a rapid decline of the quality of our life and becoming a burden on the life of others to help us living a decent life.

In order to prevent this from happening and to improve and maintain our HGH levels and muscular system as a whole, we need to signal our body that we need both the type 1, endurance, slow twitch muscle fibers as well as the type 2, strength, fast twitch muscle fibers. The method to give the body this signal is through stimulating both muscle fiber types on a regular basis through specific forms of physical activity.

The specific forms of physical activity to stimulate the two muscle fiber types are for the:

- Type 1/endurance/slow twitch muscle fibers: endurance training, also known as cardiovascular training, cardio, aerobic training or aerobics
- Type 2/strength/fast twitch muscle fibers: (high intensity) strength training, also known as resistance training, weight training and anaerobic training

Aerobic / Endurance Training

Endurance training is the name for any rhythmic activity that works large muscle groups and can be maintained for 15 to 60 minutes such as walking, riding a bike or rowing.

Endurance training is aerobic training, which means that the body uses oxygen to break down blood glucose, muscle glycogen, two or more molecules of glucose stored in the muscle cells, and fat to produce energy. It is a slow process as it takes time to transport the oxygen from the lungs through the arteries to the muscle cells. The aerobic system is great for activities that are continuous and perceived as moderate or somewhat hard.

The benefits of cardiovascular training are an increased heart activity and consequently an increased oxygen and nutrient delivery to the working muscles.

Downside is that cardiovascular training only works the type 1, endurance, slow twitch muscle fibers with the result that the type 2, strength, fast twitch muscle fibers remain unused and gradually disappear.

Your metabolic system comprises the aerobic as well as the anaerobic energy system and must therefore be trained and stimulated together. This is what happens during strength training or anaerobic training and what makes this type of training so important.

Anaerobic / High Intensity Strength Training

When an immediate release of energy is required, like in a fight or flight reaction, there is not enough time to recruit the necessary amount of oxygen for the production of energy. Therefore, the body uses an anaerobe process, a process for which the body doesn't need oxygen.

This process allows the body to do intense activity for about two minutes. This short period is a consequence of the fact that this type of energy production not only produces energy, but also a by-product called lactic acid. This lactic acid stacks up in the muscle cells and is responsible for the burning sensation in your muscles, eventually causing lactic-acidosis or muscle failure. No matter what you try at this state, it will be impossible to continue the activity you're doing which leaves you with the choice to either slow down or stop the activity. When at rest, the body converts the lactic acid back into glucose to metabolize it with the use of oxygen or aerobically.

Anaerobic training is training at a high intensity. It is a very effective way of training as the entire metabolic system including the connected muscle fibers are trained at the same time. It is a type of training however that requires working out to the limits of one's abilities to be effective.

Strength Training and The Cardiovascular System

If it is the purpose of the cardiovascular system to deliver oxygen and nutrients to the working muscles and to help remove carbon dioxide and other by-products of metabolism, then it makes only sense that the higher the stimulus and the quality of the muscular work, the greater the effect on the cardiovascular system that supports the muscular work. The next logical step is that an improved muscular strength further improves the effects on the cardiovascular system. One hand washes the other.

One of the benefits we mentioned earlier is an improved cardiovascular function. Going a little deeper on this, strength training leads to a number of beneficial effects.

-   Lower systolic blood pressure.
    This is the pressure exerted on the artery walls when the heart contracts and squeezes the blood out of the ventricles into the arteries and is the opposite of the diastolic pressure when the heart relaxes and fills itself again. When performing high intensity exercises, the secretion of the hormone adrenaline causes widening of the blood vessels in and around the working muscles. This effect helps lowering the pressure in the rest of the system.
-   A stronger heart.
    Being a muscle, a trained heart is stronger and larger than an untrained heart and therefore able to hold more blood and contract with more force. Whereas an untrained heart can hold only about 70 milliliters blood, a trained heart can hold 100 milliliters blood.
    Let's recapitulate blood circulation here. Major veins from the upper and lower body empty de-oxygenated blood into the heart's right atrium. The blood leaves the right atrium through a valve and enters the right ventricle from where it is pushed out through the lungs, where carbon dioxide will move from the blood and oxygen will move into the blood. Oxygenated blood returns to the heart into the left atrium, passes another valve and ends up in the left ventricle from where it is squeezed into the aorta, the biggest artery of the body.

The amount of blood that leaves the left ventricle of the heart is called stroke volume (SV). The amount of blood that leaves the heart in one minute is called cardiac output (Q) and is the product of stroke volume times heart rate. In other words, Q= SV x HR.

At rest your body requires about 5 liters of blood to circulate every minute. A strong heart can do the job with 60 beats but an untrained heart needs to beat 70 times for the same result. This means about 14,000 more beats during one day.

During exercise the demands for oxygen and nutrients increase. In reaction to this increased demand, both SV and HR increase in turn leading to an increased amount of blood that leaves the heart via the left ventricle every minute (Q). This process continues till it plateaus.

For example, a trained heart that beats 180 times per minute and ejects 170 milliliters per minute delivers 30,600 milliliters blood with nutrients and oxygen to the working muscles. An untrained heart beating at 180 times per minute and ejecting 100 milliliters per beat delivers only 18,000 milliliters with oxygen and nutrients to the muscles.

-   Enhanced backflow of blood to the heart.

The squeezing of the contracting muscles during exercise milks the blood back to the heart. This added to the fact that a stronger heart ejects more blood on every beat produces an enhanced coronary backflow. This effect already occurs with walking. The squeezing of the calf muscles with every step pushes blood from the lower body back toward the heart. This effect is known as the calf-pump.

The coronary arteries, located at the out- and inside of the heart walls, provide the heart with oxygen and nutrients. They are the first arteries that branch off from the aorta.

The stronger the heartbeat, the stronger will be the blood flow into the coronary arteries. More than that, when the heart relaxes after each beat to refill, part of the blood squeezed out into the aorta during the beat is sucked back into the coronary arteries at the base of the aorta. The stronger the heart the better it will be able to provide itself with sufficient oxygen and nutrients.

Completing a task such as walking up the stairs requires the activation of fewer muscles when the muscular system is in good shape. This in turn leads to a reduced demand on the cardiovascular system. To give an example, a physical weak and overweight person needs a lot of time to get at the top of the stairs and may even be panting, whereas a strong and lean person will take two steps at the time and hardly increase her or his breathing rhythm.

The Difference Between Aerobic or Endurance Workouts and Anaerobic or Strength Workouts

Many men and women tend to stay away from strength training and stick to low- and moderate impact activities such as walking the dog, working out on a treadmill, elliptical machine, bike and so on. They couldn't provide their body with a bigger disservice.

Again, our body is designed and built to work, a fact that must be respected and act upon accordingly. Working only one part of the metabolic system with cardio or endurance exercises and neglecting the other half eventually leads to health problems.

Let's line up some differences between anaerobic or strength training and aerobic or endurance training.

Endurance workouts only activate the slow twitch muscle fibers and therefore never use up the stored glycogen in the fast twitch muscle fibers. They also never completely deplete the slow twitch muscle fibers from the stored glycogen since fat is the primary energy source for low impact exercises.

As explained in "Eating for Life", the primary sources of energy during endurance workouts are carbohydrates and fat with a shifting toward fat when the workout continues for a longer time. This means that the body will only partly use up the glycogen stored in the slow twitch muscle fibers.

The fast twitch muscle fibers, the muscle fibers that contain most of the stored glycogen, will not empty their glycogen storages during endurance workouts for the simple reason that they haven't been activated.

When the slow- and fast twitch muscle fibers don't deplete themselves regularly from the stored glycogen and glucose, there is not much need for replenishment. The consequence will be that the muscle cells will eventually become less sensitive to the hormone insulin, the hormone needed to let body cells take up the glucose from the blood stream.

A loss of insulin sensitivity is one of the major causes of overweight and obesity. Most of the calories consumed after an endurance workout and during rest end up fatty acids and stored as body fat.

Strength training exercises tap into the glycogen and glucose storages of both the slow and fast twitch muscle fibers, making those muscle fibers eager to replenish themselves after a workout. Their sensitivity for insulin will increase.

This effect continues for up to 48 hours after a workout, since this is the minimum time muscle fibers need to replenish themselves after a meaningful strength-training workout.

The fact that strength training exercises stimulate the muscles to grow in strength and size results in an increased metabolic rate, which in turn leads to an increased uptake of glucose from the blood stream for the use of body functions.

Due to endurance exercises, muscles begin to waste away or atrophy because they are not used at a high enough level.

The muscle fibers that will be broken down first are the fast twitch muscle fibers. Marathon runners are a good example of this effect. Their body only maintained the muscles necessary to perform the task of running marathons and broke down the rest.

This makes sense when you keep in mind that the body is programmed to preserve energy. Maintaining and carrying around unused muscle tissue means wasting calories and is an unwanted situation that needs to be ended as quickly as possible.

Marathon runners may have managed to increase their fitness level, but they also put their health at risk in several ways. First, the constant repetitive movement of running causes a lot of wear and tear on the joints. Second, declined strength levels make them more prone to injuries. Third, decreased muscle mass leads to a decreased glycogen and glucose storing capacity in the muscle cells, which in turn increases the risk that these muscle cells become resistant to insulin.

More problems are on the rise when cells in general, and muscle cells in particular have become resistant to insulin. Under normal conditions cells use up the insulin secreted after each meal. When cells have become resistant to this hormone, part of it remains unused and causes prolonged increased insulin levels.

Insulin in itself is an inflammatory hormone and stimulates inflammatory responses in the body, for instance on the walls of the arteries and veins. As set out in the nutrition guide, inflamed areas are repaired with LDL-particles taken out of the blood stream, leading to a build-up of plaque in the blood vessels.

Elevated insulin levels keep the body in a fat storing mode. Any surplus of consumed nutrients will eventually end up as fatty acids in the fat cells and stored as body fat. Insulin has a leading role during this process.

Endurance workouts usually stretch out over a long time period and predominantly use the aerobic, oxidative metabolic system, whereas strength-training workouts activates last fairly short and use both the aerobic and anaerobic metabolic system. The consequence is that endurance workouts produce more inflammatory free radicals than strength-training workouts.

Free radicals are unstable, highly reactive molecules that lose an electron during the process of creating energy when using oxygen. It is a reaction similar to rust, the effect of a combined reaction of water and oxygen on iron.

When molecules lose an electron, they steal electrons from other molecules. These molecules then steal electrons from other molecules, thus starting a dangerous chain reaction called free radical damage.

Summarizing, strength training:

- Depletes muscles from stored glycogen
- Increases muscle mass and therefore glycogen storage
- Maintains insulin sensitivity due to the need of muscles to regularly replenish themselves after depletion
- Lowers insulin, blood pressure and cholesterol levels
- Increases metabolic rate
- Produces less free radicals due to high intense workouts and therefore shorter workouts
- Boosts heart health

The Best Of Both Worlds

The benefits of strength training don't make aerobic or endurance exercises redundant. It is never one or the other but always both. Your body is equipped with an aerobic and an anaerobic system, so both systems need to be trained to keep them in good condition. In addition, both systems never work alone, but always together.

The combination of strength and endurance is what makes it possible to perform the activities of daily life with ease and for a prolonged time.

The workouts you do should therefore consist of a combination of strength and endurance training. Combining both gives considerably more benefits than focusing on only one of the training types.

The aerobic system guarantees a constant supply of nutrients and oxygen to muscles and organs and the anaerobic system strengthens and improves the effectiveness of the aerobic system.

The First Circle of Safe and Effective Exercising, "The Fundamental Laws of Strength-Training"

To ensure a safe, effective, efficient and enjoyable training, it is essential that a strength-training program is based on six fundamental laws.

1. Enhance Joint Flexibility

Flexibility is an important condition to prevent strain, pain or injuries around the joints. Flexibility is not per se a desirable asset as both being too flexible or not flexible at all can lead to injuries. One's level of flexibility largely depends on one's genetic blueprint and must be respected when designing a training program

Goal is always enhancing flexibility more than increasing it. This means that one of the goals of a training program could be to decrease the flexibility of one joint and to increase another. Performing the exercises of a training program in a controlled full range of motion is the best guarantee to establish a healthy joint function.

2. Improve Ligament and Tendon Strength

Ligaments attach bones across a joint and tendons connect muscles to bones.

The function of ligaments is attaching bones to each other and restricting excessive motion in the joints.

The function of tendons is to transfer force from a muscle to a bone in order to facilitate movement.

It is in the joints that most injuries occur. Improving the strength of both is therefore a first condition to improve overall strength. Overloading the muscles with resistance to stimulate growth in strength and size without giving ligaments and tendons the opportunity to strengthen themselves first increases the risk of injury. Once injured, they take a long time to heal and sometimes never will for 100 percent. Effective strength training can increase ligament and tendon strength up to 20 percent.

3. Improve Core Strength

As mentioned before, the core is to support the working arms and legs and therefore often takes up the role of synergist. A weak core limits the strength and power of arms and legs, whereas a strong core allows all muscles to work longer and more effectively. The support structure of muscles running in different directions that surround the core area absorbs shocks, stabilizes the body and forms the link between arms and legs. A strength-training program must emphasize on developing core strength first before strengthening the limbs.

4. Improving Strength of Stabilizing Muscles

These muscles contract to facilitate a proper and forceful contraction of other muscles. Any muscle in the body can have this function as it depends on the performed action. A muscle can act as a prime mover or agonist, opposed to the action as antagonist or act as a stabilizer as synergist.

For example, when throwing a ball, the muscles surrounding the shoulder joint, core, knees and ankles need to fixate to provide the necessary stability in order to allow the arms to act as prime mover.

5. Multi-Joint Exercises Instead of Single Joint Exercises

Involving the use of more than one joint or one muscle group, multi joint exercises, also known as compound exercises, train various muscle groups to work together, simulating this way the activities of daily life and are the key to effective and efficient strength training.

Single joint exercises, also known as isolation exercises, emphasize on the development of a specific muscle group, as with body building. This doesn't mean that single joint exercises must always be avoided. It may for instance be necessary to perform these exercises to restore imbalances in limb strength.

6. Do What Is Needed To Achieve the Set Goals

It happens quite often that people change or quit a training program for reasons of boredom. Although it is important to regularly vary the program to keep the training challenging and motivating, changing the training program too quickly or switching to something entirely new just for the sake of doing something new or different doesn't get one closer to one's goals.

Especially during the first 8 to 12 weeks, it is important to focus consistently on building strength. After this period, it is time and even necessary to vary the exercises in order to target the muscles from different angles. From this moment on it takes every time about 4 to 6 weeks for the body to adapt to the new movements. Especially when you consider yourself a beginner, stick to each new program for this time to get the best results.

The Second Circle of Safe and Effective Exercising, "Principles of Strength Training"

The purpose of a strength-training program is to keep improving your results until you realize your goals. The principles below offer guidelines and methods to gear a training program to your specific needs. Those principles are:

1. Frequency, Intensity, Time and Type

Frequency is how often you exercise in a week.

Intensity refers to the level of difficulty of the exercises as measured in load or resistance, number of repetitions, number of sets and the rest period between the sets.

Time is how long each part of the program and the total program lasts.

Type is the choice of equipment or activity during the program.

2. Progressive Overload

This principle means that you continuously need to overload your muscles with resistance in order to keep the exercise effective. It is in fact similar to learning a new language. It can be challenging to commit new words and grammar to memory but it is the only way to improve your knowledge.

Going over words and grammar you already master won't bring you any further. Strength training works the same. It is only through a consistent and gradual increase in resistance that your muscles will become stronger. When you don't follow this principle you will eventually plateau or go backwards with your results.

3. Variety

Once you have built a basic level of strength, it is important to vary the training program on a regular basis to avoid boredom. Varying the program keeps training effective, interesting, fun and challenging for both body and mind.

Even though you feel fine with doing the same training routine every time, you have to adjust your training program at least every 4 to 6 weeks to keep body and mind guessing. Remember that your body is wired to preserve energy. As soon as it recognizes a certain pattern in the exercises you do, it begins to economize the movements to spend as less fuel as possible.

Once you are no longer a beginner with regard to strength training and have reached an intermediate or advanced, level you can even vary your training program more frequently such as every other week.

Varying a training program is not difficult. The fourth circle offers training programs with variations.

Always keep in mind not to alter a program just for the sake of doing something new. If the change of the program doesn't bring you closer to your goals then don't do it.

4. Individualization

It is important to design each training program in accordance with one's individual needs and goals as well as with one's ability, potential, rate of recovery and background. It is important to respect all the variables when designing a training program. This principle makes every training program unique. Simply following a training program that works well for somebody else doesn't mean that it will work for you in the same way.

A big misconception is that women should train differently than men. The main difference between women and men when it comes to designing training programs is the difference in strength.

Women have on average an overall strength that is about 2/3 of that of men, an upper body strength that is about 1/2 of that of men and a lower body strength that is about 3/4 of that of men. It is obvious that these facts must be taken into consideration when designing a training program but the method of designing a program for women can be similar to that of men.

Strength training is beneficial for both women and men. The rate of strength gain over a 12-week period of consistently training is similar for both sexes and sometimes even more for women than for men. In fact, women benefit most of all people of strength training as it helps to build upon bone strength and alleviates the effects of menopause.

One word of caution is appropriate for plyometric exercises. These exercises involve explosive movements such as jumping or sudden changes in direction. Because women are in general weaker means that their muscular strength around joints is in most cases weaker as well. Women therefore need to take more time to build up strength before doing plyometric exercises.

5. Specificity

After establishing a good overall strength, one can choose to adjust a training program to work toward specific goals. Preparing for a triathlon requires a different program than for a soccer tournament. Specificity enters the picture when you have passed the level of a beginner and want to focus on a certain goal. Building a strong physique always comes first to avoid an imbalanced body development and injuries. Be sure to reserve the time and the patience to do what needs to be done first and that you have developed through the four elements of fitness before doing anything else.

The Third Circle of Safe and Effective Exercising, "The Six-Step Effective Exercise Plan"

After covering the fundamental laws and principles of a training program it is time to get the conditions in place for a workout routine that will be geared toward your personal health and fitness goals and help you to achieve those goals in an safe, effective, efficient, and enjoyable way.

Essential for each training routine is consistency. It doesn't make much sense to occasionally do some exercises and forget about them when obligations or interests pop up. Doing something is of course always better than doing nothing but it hardly makes your efforts effective and efficient. You will mainly waste a lot of time and not get anywhere near your goals.

The best way to protect yourself against spinning your wheels and to get the best out of your efforts is by following the "Six Step Effective Exercise Plan" that follows the same format as the "Healthy Nutrition Plan" in Part Two "Moving for Life"

Step One, Define Your Goals

Here are six questions to answer to create a well-defined outcome.

1. Is the goal specific, realistic and positive?

Be clear about what you want to achieve. "I want to lose weight" is a good start but not enough. Be specific. How much weight do you want to lose and which parts of your body need extra attention when it comes to building or rebuilding strength?

Be sure to be realistic with regard to what you want to achieve and set a timeframe that is workable and holds you accountable at the same time. Build in time for unexpected events and delays. Things will come in your way. That's only normal, a fact of life.

Define what you *do* want, not what you *don't* want. Your subconscious mind doesn't recognize negatives and will interpret everything you think as a positive thought. For example, if you say "I don't want to be overweight", it will focus on the word "overweight" and sees that as the goal to pursue.

2. Why do I want what I want and what are the obstacles I can expect?

Does the motivation for achieving the goal come from yourself or are you stimulated by others? Your chances for success will be much bigger if the drive for realizing the desired outcome comes from within.

Do you want to achieve short-term goals such as an upcoming wedding or a vacation, or long-term goals such as maintaining an active and independent living?

Expecting that you will achieve your goals without meeting with obstacles is not realistic. In fact, obstacles are necessary for growth.

Whatever their nature, they are good. "Ah, there you are" is how you welcome and embrace them. The art is to make an inventory of the obstacles you may expect to find on your path and think of strategies to deal with them. This approach will keep your mind at ease and away from stress-reactions.

3. When will I know that I have achieved my goal?

Measure your progress by keeping track of the weights and the number of repetitions and sets you perform during your workouts. Use the workout journal you'll find in the chapter "The Full Body Workout".

To know when you have achieved intangible goals such as having more energy and looking better, ask yourself what you want to feel, hear or see when you have achieved your goal.

4. What conditions are necessary to realize my goals?

Questions you need to answer: how am I going to do it and am I going to do it by myself or with others?

5. Do I have what I need to achieve my goals?

What are the tools, skills and other recourses I now have that will help me to achieve my goals, and what more do I need?

When it comes to doing your workouts, you need to take care of practical issues such as scheduling your workouts, finding a place to do the workouts, getting equipment and comfortable workout clothing.

Also needed is developing the right attitude to workout with focus, perseverance and consistency. As always, maintain a kind, loving attitude and look at your workouts as an enjoyable and rewarding experience because it keeps your mind in a relaxed and peaceful state.

This will make it much easier to stay motivated and much easier to achieve your goals.

An aggressive attitude or looking at your workouts as a form of punishment is a sure way leads to stress and almost certainly to failure.

The fifth circle "Mastering Your Exercise Habits" gives tools and methods to develop the mindset to keep you moving forward to your goals.

6. Is the goal I want to achieve in alignment with my intentions in life?

The deeper questions you need to answer here are what is the *real* reason for my goals? How will I feel if I achieve what I want? What do I feel when I look to the future knowing that I achieved my goal? What is the best thing that could happen if I achieve my goal?

Similar to healthy nutrition, before you can actually begin defining your goals, you need to create a starting point. Describe where you are now with your weight, energy, unsupportive habits and so on. It is crucial to tune into reality. With this I mean that you have to be honest with yourself.

As mentioned earlier, no need to cut corners. Nobody is ever going to see what you write down if you don't want to. Accept whatever you write down without ever judging. Hold on to the Two-Step technique to allow only positive thoughts to remain kind and loving. No compromises here.

Therefore, spend some time on answering the questions. It is okay if you begin with a few words or short notes as you can be more elaborate any time later.

Use the "Lifestyle Change Goal-Setting Plan and Journal" you'll find at the end of this book to write down your goals following the questions above, keep track of your progress and leave comments related to challenges and successes.

Step Two, Create Your Starting Point

The purpose of a starting point is to track your progress and to obtain necessary information about your general condition and specific health issues that you have to respect when you design your training program.

Keep it simple, the following information will do to create your personal starting point.

- Ask someone to take some pictures of how you are now, wearing as less clothes as you feel comfortable with
- measure your body length
- weigh yourself
- measure your waist and hip girth
- write down your general energy levels throughout the day, and
- write down how you feel about yourself and what thoughts, beliefs and habits are holding you back setting up a regular exercise routine.

Set up an appointment with your doctor if you meet any of the following criteria:

- you are over age 60 and not accustomed to vigorous exercise
- you have a family history of premature coronary heart disease under 55 years of age
- you frequently have pains or pressure in the left or mid chest area, left neck, shoulder or arm during or immediately after exercise
- you often feel faint or have spells of severe dizziness, or you experience extreme breathlessness after mild exertion

- your doctor has said that your blood pressure is too high, or you don't have your blood pressure measured on a regular basis
- your doctor has said that you have heart trouble, that you have a heart murmur, or that you have had a heart attack
- your doctor has said that you have bone or joint problems, such as arthritis
- you have a medical condition that might need special attention in an exercise program

Use your common sense. Always see your doctor if you are in doubt.

Step Three, Design Your Program

The three basic elements your training program consists of are healthy nutrition, a combined strength- and cardio or endurance workout program and anchors that keep you on track toward your goals.

- Healthy nutrition

What you need to know to get and keep yourself on track with regard to healthy nutrition is covered in "Eating for Life". Be sure to have that in place before you begin a training program. Nutrition is the foundation of all health and fitness and it really makes no sense to start building a heathy, strong physique without providing your body with the right fuel and building materials coming from healthy nutrition.

- A combined strength and cardio or endurance workout program

You will find a workout program in the next chapter. Use this program as your personal starting point.

- Anchors that keep you on track

What works to get and keep you on track with nutrition works similar for your training program. Find anchors that help you with establishing a continuous training program without interruptions.

Anchors to put in place:

Block time in your agenda to workout. An hour workout only takes up about six percent of the sixteen hours of a day you are awake.

Keep track of your results by keeping a "Weekly Workout Journal". Nothing is more stimulating and motivating than following your progress. Write down the exercises you do, the number of sets, the number of repetitions and your overall workout time. Keeping track of your results also gives you important information to see when it is time to change your program. You'll find a template "Weekly Workout Journal" in this book.

Find people you can train with or, if you prefer to train on your own, go to places where you find like-minded people. Follow successful people and avoid people and places that make it difficult or even impossible to achieve your goals.

Tell family and friends about your goals and that you expect them to support you. Commit yourself to sending them a picture of yourself every month with the latest results of your training program and body weight.

Keep educating yourself once you get the hang of healthy nutrition and safe and effective exercising. Find information wherever you can and connect to like-minded people. It is rewarding and you can be an example and support for other people who also want to improve their quality of life.

Apply the Two-Step meditation practice to get and keep you on track toward your goals. In the fifth circle "Mastering Your Exercise Habits", we'll go over the tools and the techniques.

Step 4, Take Action

Action is all about implementing the programs. If you have your training and nutrition programs in place including the anchors that will keep you going but don't take the necessary action then everything remains the same.

Again, this is the point where the majority of the information you read about nutrition and exercising tell you goodbye with a closing statement sounding like: "The start of a new program, any new program, is never an easy thing to do. It takes about 21 days to cement new habits into your life style, but then routine kicks in and things will go easier. The art is not to let get anything in your way to achieve your goals. Be persistent."

There is of course nothing wrong with these words but the point is that these words forget the role the conscious and subconscious mind play in building a regular workout routine. It is the metaphor about the runway again. It is impossible to expect from an aircraft to take off when it has its engines going and all its systems checked but doesn't have a runway to gain the necessary speed for take-off.

You know where I'm going to. Through applying the Two-Step technique, you can get the necessary speed to gain momentum, make regular exercising part of your life and make life more enjoyable.

It may still sound a bit abstract at this point and that is fine. The fifth circle will provide you with the insights, tools and methods to make regular exercising a natural part of your life.

Simply keep reading through the information that follows and gently dismiss the automatic reactions from your subconscious mind that may hold feelings of doubt and prejudices. They *are* not you. You only *have* them.

Let's continue.

Step Five, Focus – Action – Reflection

What works for healthy nutrition works similarly for safe and effective exercising. Remaining aware of where you are, what you think, feel, see and do throughout the day offers you the opportunity to grab the conductor's stick. This means that you consciously use your conscious mind to decide whether what you experience is consistent with your intentions and goals, or that it is time to make some adjustments.

Applying the routine of Focus – Action – Reflection helps you to keep peace of mind and improve your results. Be aware of the moment, accept any situation you run into as is, look at your past successes, reflect upon the challenges facing you and determine the best action to take.

At the end of this book you'll find the checklist "Optimizing Results Training Program" to help you with the process of reviewing the results of your training routine.

This checklist goes by all the five individual circles and their important topics and helps you to determine whether there is room for improvement.

The Fourth Circle of Safe and Effective Exercising, "The Full Body Workout"

Step three of the "Six-Step Effective Exercise Plan" mentioned designing a combined strength and endurance-training program. In this chapter, you will find a full body workout you can start with to make the first steps toward improving your fitness.

Stay on the safe side when you make your start. Proper technique always comes first. Compromising form to overcome a resistance is sure-way to injury. Avoid this situation at all times.

The Workout

Over the next pages we go through a workout you can do anywhere. The workout takes up 45 to 60 minutes and most of the exercises can be performed using your own bodyweight. Do the workout without weights when you consider yourself a beginner. As soon as you have made yourself familiar with the exercises and want to make the workout more challenging, you can do the workout using free weights such as dumbbells or barbells.

A full body workout ideally starts with the bigger muscle groups, followed by the smaller muscle groups.

The sequence of the muscle groups covered in this workout is as follows,

1. Warm-up
2. Legs, Squats
3. Chest, Push-Ups, Barbell or Dumbbell Presses
4. Back, Row, Row-Clean and Press, Good Morning Lift
5. Arms, Biceps
6. Arms, Triceps Extension, Close Grip Press
7. Legs, Lunges
8. Shoulders
9. Core
10. Cool-down

You'll do the legs in this workout twice for two reasons. First, they are bigger compared to the other muscle groups and second, working out the legs requires involvement of major stabilizing muscle groups and underlying smaller muscle fibers in the body.

Because of the importance of a proper warm-up prior to the workout, and a cool-down at the end of the workout I made both part of the workout.

Workout Guide lines

1. The exercises of the workout are performed in 2 to 3 sets with 8 to 12 repetitions per set for the upper body and 16 repetitions for the lower body because of the bigger muscle groups.

2. The last repetitions of each set must be tough to finish, but not so difficult that you have to compromise form.

3. If you can do more than 12 repetitions per set for the upper body or 16 for the lower body you're working more on endurance than on building strength. Increase the weight when you can do more than the mentioned repetitions with proper form.

4. Keep in mind to be sure that you perform the exercises with proper form before you increase the weight.

5. Start the exercises with slow movements; 2 to 4 to counts up and 2 to 4 counts down or even slower. Going slow has several advantages over faster movements:

First, you've the time to check whether you're performing the exercises correctly.

Second, you have better control during the movement.

Third, slow and controlled movements provide the best stimulus for your muscles to grow in strength and size.

Fourth, if there are issues in joints or muscles, you have the time to work around those issues or to stop the exercise before injuring yourselves.

Fifth, slow movements avoid momentum or mass x velocity or swing, which makes the movements more challenging as a result of which it possible to work with lower weights.

6. Important is to start off on the easy-side and work up to avoid injury. If you push yourself to the limit on the first day, you'll be dealing with more muscle soreness than necessary for days and that's obviously not going to help you toward your health and fitness goals.

7. Drink enough prior to the workout and between the exercises. Forget about those energy drinks loaded with sugar and chemicals. Plain water is best.

8. Vary your workout regularly. It is time to make some changes after doing the same program 4 to 6 times. Don't allow your body to get used to a certain routine. It will start economizing which means that you will make less progress. So challenge your body in several ways by changing up the program.

9. Consider your experience when planning the amount of time for a workout. Start with a short duration, like 5 or 10 minutes, when you are a beginner, and increase your workout time gradually every week to between 45 and 60 minutes.

10. Workout twice a week with 2 to 3 resting days between the workouts. This is a guideline. Listen to your body, learn to interpret the signals or body responses during the days that follow your workout and respect them.

Keep Track of Your Results in a Workout Journal

A workout journal is a motivational tool and provides you with important information about your progress and when it is time to change the program. You can use the template below.

Most of the exercises in the workout journal mention variations. The first exercise for the legs mentions the squat in a wide stance, a shoulder width stance and a narrow stance. Choose the shoulder width stance for your first workouts. After a few weeks, when you have become familiar with one of the variations, you can begin to make combinations such as three sets consisting of one set of each of the variations. You'll find more suggestions for variations later in this chapter.

Workout Journal Week...................

Exercises	Variations	Weight(s)	Sets	Reps	Comments
Warm-up					
Legs	Squat Wide stance	.......X.......	....	X	
	Squat shoulder width stance	.......X.......	....	X	
	Squat narrow stance	.......X.......	....	X	
Chest	Regular Pushup	.......X.......	....	X	
	Modified Pushup	.......X.......	....	X	
	Chest Press	.......X.......	....	X	
Back	Row	.......X.......	....	X	

	Row-Clean and Press	.......X.......	....	X	
	Good Morning	.......X.......	....	X	
Biceps	Biceps Curl	.......X.......	....	X	
	Concentration Curl	.......X.......	....	X	
Triceps	Extension	.......X.......	....	X	
	Close Grip Bench Press	.......X.......	....	X	
	Dumbbell Kick Back		....	X	
Legs	Lunges	.......X.......	....	X	
Shoulders	Rear deltoids	2 X..........	....	X	
	Lateral raise	2 X..........	....	X	
	Front raise	2 X.......	....	X	
	Shoulder Press	2 X.......	....	X	
Core	Sit up		....	X	
	Crunch		....	X	
	Leg raise		....	X	
	Oblique crunch		....	X	
	Oblique side bent		....	X	
Cool down					

The Warm-Up, the Beginning of Every Workout

I can't emphasize enough the importance of a proper warm-up. A warm-up is necessary to prepare yourself both physically and mentally for the workout. The physical part of the warm-up is to adjust blood flow, warm up the nervous system and the muscles. The mental part of the warm-up is to bring your undivided attention to the exercises you will perform.

In general, don't do too difficult about what movements to choose for a warm-up. Think of the activity you're planning to do and simply perform a lighter version. Walk before you jog and jog before you run, and so on.

A word of caution, don't try to warm up by stretching your muscles. Putting a force at the extreme range of motion of a cold muscle only maximizes the risk of injury. You warm up your body with muscle contractions, not with muscle stretches for the simple reason that the former produces the necessary body heat, the latter doesn't.

To warm up for this workout you can do the following movements. March in place for about 1 minute while rolling your shoulders backwards and performing upward, front and side arm reaches. Follow up with 10 lunges, 10 dead lifts and 10 squats.

If you're not yet familiar with the movements, begin with some light jogging in place with simple arm and core movements for about 3 to 5 minutes.

If you want, you can use light weights, a barbell with plates or no weights at all. All choices are fine since it is only meant to warm up.

The image below indicates the location of the main muscles worked during the exercises.

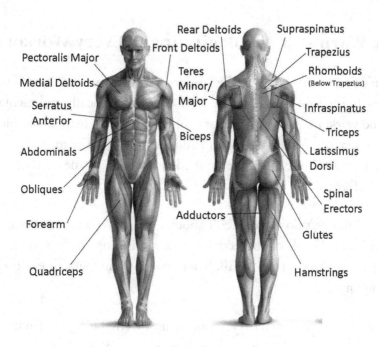

The Muscular System

Human Body Back/Front with Major Muscle Groups

Legs, Squats

Muscles Involved

Quadriceps, glutes, hamstrings, adductors, spinal erectors and abdominals

Start Position

Feet shoulder width apart, toes slightly pointing out, knees slightly bent and upright upper body.

Execution:

- Lower your body by bending your knees as if taking a seat
- Stick your glutes backwards and point your chest forward, keep your feet flat on the floor
- Bend your knees until your thighs are parallel to the floor
- Squeeze your glutes and push through the balls and the heels of your feet while you straighten your legs to return to the start position
- Don't lock out your joints, keep your knees slightly bent
- Keep your spine straight and your head up
- Be sure you can wiggle your toes at all times
- Inhale during the downward phase and exhale on the way up.

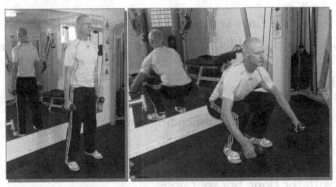

Start and End Position   Mid Position

Legs, Squat Exercise

Variation

Perform the exercise with the starting position in a narrow or wide stance

Sets / Reps / Rest

Do 2 or 3 sets of 12 to 16 repetitions with 30 seconds rest between the sets. Perform the downward movement in 4 counts and the upward movement in 2 counts.

Weight

Choose a weight or weights heavy enough to make it difficult to complete the last repetitions but not so difficult that you have to compromise your form.

Chest, Push-Ups

Muscles involved

Pectoralis major, front deltoids and triceps

Start Position

Hands flat on the floor at shoulder level, slightly wider than shoulder width, legs straight and feet together, toes tucked under your feet.

Execution

- Lower your body by bending your arms while keeping your back straight
- Look a bit forward, chin and chest must make the first contact with the floor, not your nose
- Straighten your arms as you push your body away from the floor

- Don't bend or arch your upper or lower back when you push up
- Inhale during the downward phase and exhale on the way up.

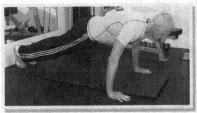 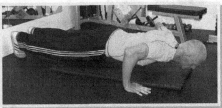

Start and End Position   Mid Position

Chest, Pushup Exercise

Variation 1

Do the modified push-up when you are not strong enough in your chest and arms with the start position on your knees instead of your toes.

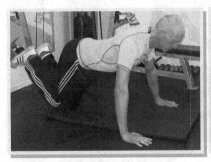 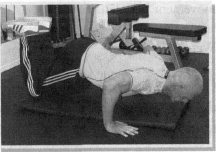

Start and End Position   Mid Position

Chest, Pushup Exercise, Variation, Modified Pushup

Variation 2

While lying on your back, use free weights or a barbell with plates

- Start at chest level, midline chest, hands shoulder width, palms facing forward
- Press the weights till elbows almost lock out
- Lower the weights or the barbell down to midline chest

- Keep your core tight, don't arch your back

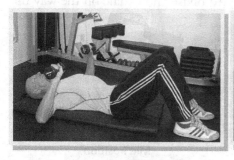 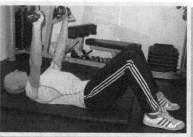

| Start and End Position | Mid Position |

Chest, Pushup Exercise, Variation Dumbbell Press

Sets / Reps / Rest

Do 2 or 3 sets of 8 to 12 repetitions with 30 seconds rest between the sets. Perform the downward movement in 4 counts and the upward movement in 2 counts.

Weight

Choose a weight or weights heavy enough to make it difficult to complete the last repetitions but not so difficult that you have to compromise your form.

Back, Row

Muscles involved

Latissimus dorsi, spinal erectors, trapezius, rhomboids and rear deltoids

Start position

Set your feet shoulder width apart with knees slightly bent, toes slightly pointing out and upper body upright. Hold the weights or the bar at shoulder width in an overhand grip.

Execution

- Bend forward at your waist until at an angle of 45 degrees to the floor while keeping your upper body straight by keeping your shoulders back and your chest pointing forward
- Pull the weights or the bar toward your stomach
- Lower the arms to the extended position
- Inhale during the downward phase and exhale on the way up

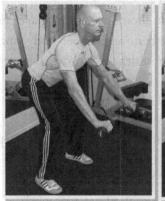 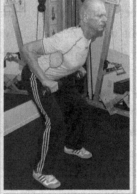

Start and End Position   Mid Position

Back, Row Exercise

Sets / Reps / Rest

Do 2 or 3 sets of 8 to 12 repetitions with 30 seconds rest between the sets. Retract elbows in 2 counts and extend arms in 4 counts.

Weight

Choose a weight or weights heavy enough to make it difficult to complete the last repetitions but not so difficult that you have to compromise your form.

Back, Row - Clean and Press

Muscles involved

Latissimus dorsi, trapezius, deltoids, spinal erectors, rhomboids and upper pectoralis

Start position

Set your feet a little wider than shoulder width apart, toes slightly pointing out with knees slightly bent and upper body upright. Hold the weights or the bar at shoulder width.

Execution

- Bend forward at your waist until at an angle of 45 degrees to the floor while keeping your upper body straight by keeping your shoulders back and your chest pointing forward
- Pull the weights or the bar toward your stomach
- Lower the arms back to the extended position
- Come back in the upright position
- Pull weights or bar upward, keeping them close to your body, to chin level and raising the arms as high as possible
- Tuck the elbows in and under the weight, flip the weight, bend your knees at the same time and use arms and shoulders to press the weight up over your head
- Reverse the motion by lowering the arms, flipping back down the weights while bending the knees again a bit
- Lower your arms, keeping the weight close to your body

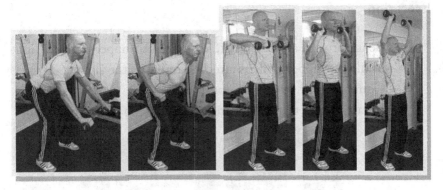

Start Mid and End Position

Back, Row – Clean and Press Exercise

Sets / Reps / Rest

Do 2 to 3 sets of 8 to 12 repetitions in a slow and controlled motion with 30 seconds rest between the sets.

Weight

Choose a weight or weights heavy enough to make it difficult to complete the last repetitions, but not so difficult that you have to compromise your form.

Back, Good Morning Lift

Muscles involved

Spinal erectors, latissimus dorsi, glutes and hamstrings

Start position

Set your feet a little wider than shoulder width apart with knees slightly bent, toes slightly pointing out and upper body upright. Hold the weights against your chest or the barbell across the shoulders.

Execution

- Bend forward at your waist, keeping your upper body straight until your upper body is almost parallel to the floor
- Come back in the upright position
- Inhale during the downward phase and exhale on the way up

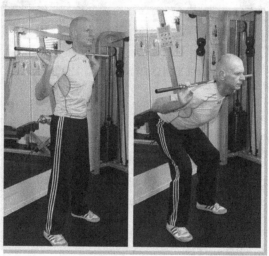

Start and End Position   Mid Position

Back, Good Morning Lift exercise

Sets / Reps / Rest

Do 2 to 3 sets of 8 to 12 repetitions in a slow and controlled motion with 30 seconds rest between the sets.

Weight

Choose a weight or weights heavy enough to make it difficult to complete the last repetitions, but not so difficult that you have to compromise your form.

Arms, Biceps

Muscles involved

Biceps, front deltoids and forearms

Start position

Set your feet a little wider than shoulder width apart with knees slightly bent, toes slightly pointing out and upper body upright. Keep your arms outside your hips and hold the weights or the barbell in an underhand grip.

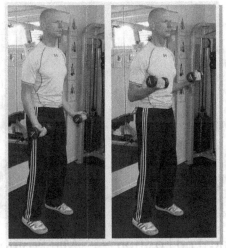

Start and End Position   Mid Position

Arms, Standing Biceps Curl Exercise

Execution

- Bend your elbows and curl up the arms up to shoulder level
- Keep your elbows close to your side without digging them into your core for support, don't let them come forward or go backward
- Keep your core tight, don't swing
- Inhale during the downward phase and exhale on the way up

Variation

Concentration curl

- Sit on a bench or a chair, legs apart, let one upper arm rest against the inner thigh. Hold a weight in an underhand grip and keep your back straight.

Execution:

- Curl the arm holding the weight toward the shoulder while holding the knee with the other hand for support.

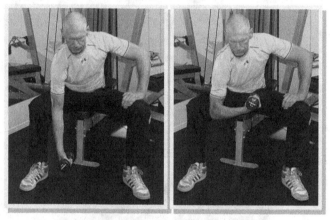

Start and End Position   Mid Position

Arms, concentration biceps curl exercise

Sets / Reps / Rest

Do 2 or 3 sets of 8 to 12 repetitions with 30 seconds rest between the sets. Perform the downward movement in 4 counts and the upward movement in 2 counts.

Weight

Choose a weight or weights heavy enough to make it difficult to complete the last repetitions but not so difficult that you have to compromise your form.

Arms, Triceps Extension

Muscles involved

Triceps, pectoralis major, deltoids and forearms

Start position

Lying on your back on the floor or a flat bench, hold free weights or a barbell in a narrow overhand grip above your chest and keep your arms and elbows in line with your shoulders.

Execution

- Bend the arms at the elbows and lower the weights/barbell till they almost touch the forehead
- Keep your elbows together in line with your shoulders, don't let them sway outward
- Push the weights or barbell upward till your elbows almost lock out
- Inhale during the downward phase and exhale on the way up

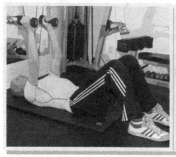 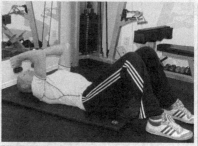

Start and End Position   Mid Position

Arms, Triceps Extension Exercise

Sets / Reps / Rest

Do 2 or 3 sets of 8 to 12 repetitions with 30 seconds rest between the
sets. Perform the downward movement in 4 counts and the upward
movement in 2 counts.

Weight

Choose a weight or weights heavy enough to make it difficult to complete
the last repetitions but not so difficult that you have to compromise your
form.

Arms, Triceps, Close Grip Press

Muscles involved

Triceps, pectoralis major and front deltoids

Start position

Lying on your back on the floor or a flat bench, hold free weights or a
barbell in a narrow overhand grip above your chest and keep your arms
in line with your shoulders.

Execution

- Lower the weights back down to midline chest
- Push the weights or barbell straight up until your elbows almost lock out,
- Inhale during the downward phase and exhale on the way up

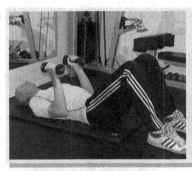 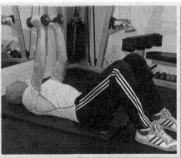

Start and End Position   Mid Position

Arms, Triceps Extension Close Grip Press Exercise

Sets / Reps / Rest

Do 2 or 3 sets of 8 to 12 repetitions with 30 seconds rest between the sets. Perform the downward movement in 4 counts and the upward movement in 2 counts.

Weight

Choose a weight or weights heavy enough to make it difficult to complete the last repetitions but not so difficult that you have to compromise your form.

Arms, Triceps, Dumbbell Kick Back

Muscles involved

Triceps, pectoralis major and front deltoids

Start position

Feet shoulder width apart, knees slightly bent and a straight upper body.

Execution

- Bend forward at the waist and support your upper body by resting your free hand on your knee or on a bench or a chair
- Hold your upper arm parallel to the floor and your elbow close to your side at a 90 degree angle
- Hold the weight in a neutral grip, thumb forward, and raise the weight upward till your arms are fully extended
- Inhale during the downward phase and exhale on the way up

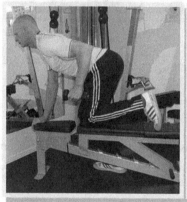 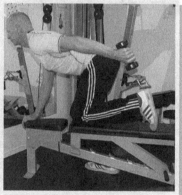

Start and End Position   Mid Position

Arms, Triceps Extension Kick Back Exercise

Sets / Reps / Rest

Do 2 or 3 sets of 8 to 12 repetitions with 30 seconds rest between the sets. Perform the downward movement in 4 counts and the upward movement in 2 counts.

Weight

Choose a weight or weights heavy enough to make it difficult to complete the last repetitions but not so difficult that you have to compromise your form.

Legs, Lunges

Muscles involved

Quadriceps, glutes, hamstrings and adductors

Start position

Feet shoulder width apart, knees slightly bent and upright upper body, while holding weights in your hands or resting a barbell across your shoulders.

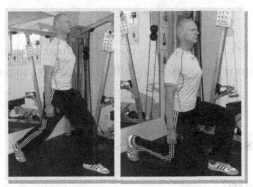

Start and End Position   Mid Position

Legs, Lunges Exercise

Execution

- Take a big step forward and bend the knee until your front upper leg is parallel to the floor and the upper leg of the other leg is in vertical position. Don't let the knee of your rear leg touch the floor.
- Return to the start position but keep the knee of your front leg slightly bent
- Don't let your knee of your front leg come in front of your ankle and keep your upper body upright
- Inhale during the downward phase and exhale on the way up

Sets / Reps / Rest

Do 2 or 3 sets of 12 to 16 repetitions with 30 seconds rest between the sets. Perform the downward movement in 4 counts and the upward movement in 2 counts.

Weight

Choose a weight or weights heavy enough to make it difficult to complete the last repetitions but not so difficult that you have to compromise your form.

Shoulders, Rear Deltoids

Muscles involved

Front deltoids, trapezius, rhomboids, teres minor and major and infraspinatus.

Start position

Feet shoulder width apart, knees slightly bent, toes slightly pointing out and upright upper body while holding weights in your hands.

Execution

- Bend forward at the waist until in a 45 degree angle and keep upper body straight by pointing your chest forward
- Turn your elbows slightly outward and pull them back keeping your elbows high
- Bring your arms in front position and repeat
- Work from your shoulders and keep your neck free of tension
- Inhale during the downward phase and exhale on the way up

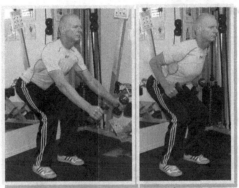

Start and End Position   Mid Position

Shoulders, Rear Deltoids Exercise

Sets / Reps / Rest

Do 2 or 3 sets of 8 to 12 repetitions with 30 seconds rest between the sets. Perform the downward movement in 4 counts and the upward movement in 2 counts.

Weight

Choose a weight or weights heavy enough to make it difficult to complete the last repetitions but not so difficult that you have to compromise your form.

Shoulders, Medial Deltoids

Muscles involved

Medial deltoids, trapezius, and supraspinatus

Start position

Feet shoulder width apart, knees slightly bent, toes slightly pointing out and upright upper body while holding weights in your hands with the thumbs forward.

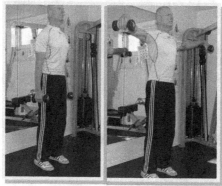

Start and End Position   Mid Position

Shoulders, Medial Deltoids Exercise

Execution

- Raise arms to the side till the arms are at shoulder level
- Work from your shoulders and keep your neck free of tension
- Lower weights back to the hips and repeat
- Inhale during the upward phase and exhale on the way up

Sets / Reps / Rest

Do 2 or 3 sets of 8 to 12 repetitions with 30 seconds rest between the sets. Perform the downward movement in 4 counts and the upward movement in 2 counts.

Weight

Choose a weight or weights heavy enough to make it difficult to complete the last repetitions but not so difficult that you have to compromise your form.

Shoulders, Front Deltoids

Muscles involved

Front deltoids, trapezius and pectoralis.

Start position

Feet shoulder width apart, knees slightly bent, toes slightly pointing out and upright upper body.

Execution

- Raise arms to the front till the arms are at shoulder level
- Lower the weights back to the hips and repeat
- Work from your shoulders and keep your neck free of tension
- Inhale during the downward phase and exhale on the way up

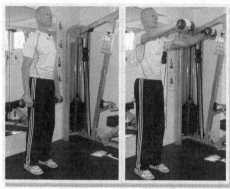

Start and End Position   Mid Position

Shoulders, Front Deltoids Exercise

Sets / Reps / Rest

Do 2 or 3 sets of 8 to 12 repetitions with 30 seconds rest between the sets. Perform the downward movement in 4 counts and the upward movement in 2 counts.

Weight

Choose a weight or weights heavy enough to make it difficult to complete the last repetitions but not so difficult that you have to compromise your form.

Shoulders, Shoulder Press

Muscles involved:

Front and medial deltoids, trapezius, triceps and pectorals

Start position

Sit or stand, feet shoulder width apart, knees slightly bent, toes slightly pointing out and upright upper body while holding weights or a barbell in an overhand grip.

Execution

- Pull weights or bar in a wide grip upward, holding them close to your body, to chin level and raising the arms as high as possible
- Tuck the elbows in and under the weight, flip the weight, bend your knees at the same time and use arms and shoulders to push the weight up over your head
- Lower the arms till they are at upper chest level and push upward again till the arms are fully extended
- Work from your shoulders and keep your neck free of tension
- Inhale during the downward phase and exhale on the way up

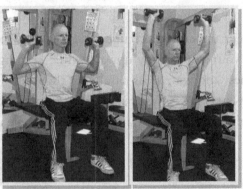

Start and End Position   Mid Position

Shoulders, Shoulder Press Exercise

Sets / Reps / Rest

Do 2 or 3 sets of 8 to 12 repetitions with 30 seconds rest between the sets. Perform the downward movement in 4 counts and the upward movement in 2 counts.

Weight

Choose a weight or weights heavy enough to make it difficult to complete the last repetitions but not so difficult that you have to compromise your form.

Core, Floor Abdominal Crunch

Muscles involved

Abdomen, obliques and serratus anterior.

Start position

Lie flat on the floor, knees bent, feet flat on the floor, fingers behind the ears and your chin off your chest.

Execution

- Keep your upper body straight and focus on your abdominals to pull your upper body upward while keeping your chin off your chest and your arms parallel to the floor
- Lower your body till your shoulders almost touch the floor
- Inhale during the downward phase and exhale on the way up

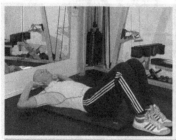 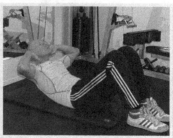

Start and End Position   Mid Position

Floor, Abdominal Crunch Exercise

Sets / Reps / Rest

Do 2 or 3 sets of 8 to 12 repetitions with 30 seconds rest between the sets. Perform the downward movement in 2 counts and the upward movement in 2 counts.

Weight

You can hold a weight against your chest during the exercise. Choose a weight heavy enough to make it difficult to complete the last repetitions but not so difficult that you have to compromise your form.

Core, Floor Abdominal Crunch, Knees Bent

Muscles involved

Abdomen and obliques

Start position

Lie flat on the floor, hips bent at 90 degrees, fingers behind the ears and chin off your chest.

Execution

- Raise your shoulders, crunching your chest forward while keeping your chin off your chest and your arms parallel to the floor and keeping your lower back in contact with the floor
- Lower your body till your shoulders almost touch the floor and repeat
- Inhale during the downward phase and exhale on the way up

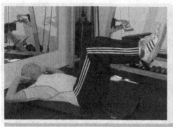 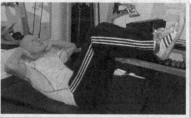

Start and End Position   Mid Position

Floor, Abdominal Crunch Exercise, Knees Bent

Sets / Reps / Rest

Do 2 or 3 sets of 8 to 12 repetitions with 30 seconds rest between the sets. Perform the downward movement in 2 counts and the upward movement in 2 counts.

Weight

You can hold a weight against your chest during the exercise. Choose a weight heavy enough to make it difficult to complete the last repetitions but not so difficult that you have to compromise your form.

Core, Leg Raise

Muscles involved

Lower abdomen and obliques.

Start position

Lie flat on the floor, legs extended, hands with the palms facing downward half under your glutes, chin off your chest.

Execution

- Raise your legs while keeping your lower back in contact with the floor
- Lower your legs till your heels almost touch the floor and repeat
- Inhale during the downward phase and exhale on the way up

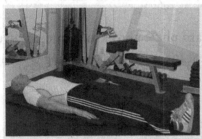 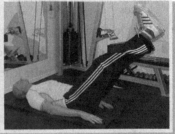

Start and End Position   Mid Position

Core, leg raise exercise

Sets / Reps / Rest

Do 2 or 3 sets of 8 to 12 repetitions with 30 seconds rest between the sets. Perform the downward movement in 4 counts and the upward movement in 2 counts.

Core, Oblique Crunch

Muscles involved

Abdomen and obliques

Start position

Lie on your right side on the floor, hips bent at 90 degrees, left hand behind your head.

Execution

- Lift your upper body and move your right shoulder toward your knees while keeping your chin off your chest and your arms flared out
- Lower your body back to the floor
- Lift your upper body and move your left shoulder toward your knees
- Inhale during the downward phase and exhale on the way up
- Lower your body and repeat the movement bringing your right shoulder toward your knees

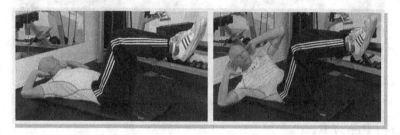

Start and End Position   Mid Position

Core, Oblique Crunch Exercise

Sets / Reps / Rest

Do 2 or 3 sets of 8 to 12 repetitions to each side with 30 seconds rest between the sets. Perform the downward movement in 2 counts and the upward movement in 2 counts.

Weight:

You can hold a weight against your chest during the exercise. Choose a weight heavy enough to make it difficult to complete the last repetitions but not so difficult that you have to compromise your form.

Core, Oblique, Side Crunch

Muscles involved

Serratus anterior, obliques and abdomen

Start position

Feet shoulder width apart, knees slightly bent, upright upper body, holding a weight in your right hand and your left hand behind your head.

Execution

- Bend upper body to the left side, lowering the weight toward your knee
- Come back in upright position, contracting the right oblique muscles and repeat
- Inhale during the downward phase, exhale on the way up
- Repeat the movement for the other side after completing one set

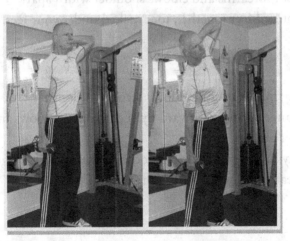

Start and End Position   Mid Position

Core, Oblique Side Crunch Exercise

Sets / Reps / Res

Do 2 or 3 sets of 8 to 12 repetitions with 30 seconds rest between the sets. Perform the downward movement in 2 counts and the upward movement in 2 counts.

Weight

Choose a weight heavy enough to make it difficult to complete the last repetitions but not so difficult that you have to compromise your form.

Core, Plank

Muscles involved

Serratus anterior, obliques, abdomen, hamstrings, glutes, spinal erector, latissimus dorsi and front deltoids.

Start position

Lean on your forearms and elbows shoulder width apart, back straight, legs straight and feet together, toes tucked under your feet.

Execution

- Stay in this position for 30 seconds or longer
- Lean a bit more forward by tucking your elbows more toward your abs
- Stay in this position for another 30 seconds or longer
- Breathe normally during the exercise

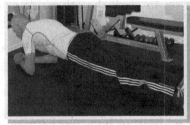 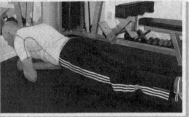

Start and End Position   Mid Position

Core, Plank Exercise

Weight

To make the exercise more challenging, lift your legs alternately during the exercise.

Variation

Side plank

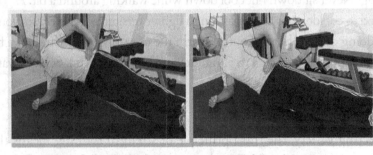

Start and End Position Mid Position

Image: Core, side plank exercise

Execution:

- Come on one side while leaning on one forearm and elbow
- Keep your core straight and tight
- Lower hip to the floor and bring it back up as high as you can

- Turn 180 degrees after each set to work the other side of the body
- Breathe normally during the exercise

Sets / Reps / Rest

Do 2 or 3 sets of 8 to 12 repetitions with 30 seconds rest between the sets. Perform the downward movement in 2 counts and the upward movement in 2 counts.

Weight

To make the exercise more challenging, lift your leg during the exercise.

Cooldown

The purpose of a cooldown is to allow your heart rate to go gradually back to levels that belong to normal daily activities. Most importantly is to keep moving. Never sit down but cool down while walking around a bit. A good method to cooldown is by performing a lighter version of the exercises you've been doing during the workout. Perform the exercises slowly through a full range of motion for about 3 to 5 minutes and be sure to drink enough water.

Varying Your Workouts

Respecting variety, the third principle of strength training means that you have to spice up your workouts regularly to keep the workouts challenging and inspiring for both body and mind. Some suggestions:

- Begin with simple variations such as choosing for one of the variations mentioned in the Workout journal.
- Increase the weights when you can do more than 8 to 12 repetitions and 16 for the legs with proper form.
- Vary the speed of the movements. Instead of doing the downward in 4 counts and the upward phase in 2 counts, you can slow down or speed up the phases. Some examples are,

Downward phase	Upward phase
4 counts	2 counts
4 counts	1 count
1 count	4 counts
1 count	1 count

And so on. This method gives you already 16 variations to play with. Be careful when doing the 1-count up, 1-count downward phases since they require extra core and joint stability in order to maintain proper form.

Research learned that performing the exercises at a speed of 2 counts during the contracting phase or concentric phase and 4 counts stretching or eccentric phase is most effective to build strength, so mainly focus on this speed variation.

Having said this, varying in speed trains the neuromuscular system to accommodate slow as well as fast movements, which is important since you also constantly alter the speed of your movements during activities of daily life.

Some more suggestions for variations:

Extend the downward or upward phases of the exercises beyond 4 counts. Challenge yourself to extend the counting to 6, 10 or 20 per phase. Find out how far you can push yourself without compromising form.

Use only one weight instead of two when performing the exercises. This way of training requires extra core involvement, especially from the underlying smaller muscle fibers.

Vary the resting time between the sets. Start for instance with 45 seconds rest between the sets and take off 5 seconds of the rest periods between the sets every following week.

Change up the sequence of the exercises. As mentioned before, a full body workout ideally begins with the bigger muscle groups. However, once familiar with all the exercises and the routine, there is nothing wrong with changing up the sequence of the exercises.

The workout consists of two subgroups, the first subgroup being "The Big Three", legs, chest and back, and the second subgroup the rest of the exercises, which mainly work the smaller muscle groups, aside from the legs.

"The Big Three" works all the major muscle groups of the body so it is best to keep changes in the sequence of these exercises within this first subgroup and any other changes in the second subgroup.

"The Big Three", A Mini-Workout

The fact that the exercises of "The Big Three" work all the major muscle groups of the body makes it possible to do only these exercises and still work your entire body. This can serve as a great alternative for those occasions that you do not have the time to do the entire workout.

See this mini workout only as a way to squeeze in some exercises to boost your metabolism or to loosen up your body after a period of inactivity but don't let it replace a regular workout as it won't give you all the benefits of a complete workout.

Keep Your Focus on Working Your Entire Metabolic System

Whenever you do a workout, be sure that it is effective and that you always work your entire metabolic system, in other words, work both your slow and fast twitch muscle fibers and keep the resting periods between the sets short.

Any type of workout at low to moderate impact level only works the slow twitch or endurance muscle fibers and does not push your neuromuscular system nor your cardiorespiratory system or your energy system. Reserve the low to moderate impact activities for the recovery days between two workouts.

The simple signs by which you can tell you are working out effectively is when you are out of breath, build up a sweat and feel your muscles burn. This way you are pushing your limits, which is your ultimate goal.

A question I sometimes get is "How can I do a workout effectively when I'm not at home where I have my weights and can't go to a gym?"

The answer: perform the exercises either really slow or very fast.

Slow movements eliminate momentum, the product of mass x velocity, which makes an exercise much more challenging. Try for yourself. Do 10 squats or push-ups with a 2 count downward and upward phase, take a few minutes rest and then do only one squat or push-up with a 10 count downward- and upward phase. You will feel the difference.

Fast and explosive movements on the other hand require the activation of fast twitch or strength muscle fibers, which makes an exercise also very effective. Perform the exercise as fast as you can, rest for 30 seconds and repeat.

A word of caution though, a fast and explosive performance of exercises requires perfect form, strong joints and a strong core. Apply this form of training only if you feel strong and secure enough. Women in particular need to take more time to strengthen their ligaments and tendons before engaging themselves in this type of training. This is particularly the case for plyometric exercises that include jumping and sudden changes in directions.

Optimize Your Breathing

About 80 percent of the people breathe incorrectly. It makes a big difference whether you breathe through your nose or through your mouth. Breathing through your nose is best for the following reasons:

- Air is warmed and moisturized before it enters your lungs. It is easier for your lungs to extract oxygen from moisturized air than from dry air
- The tiny hairs lining the inside of your nose filter out bacteria, dust and other particles that shouldn't reach your lungs
- Information about the air you breathe in through your nose is passed on to your brain for processing
- Your nose and sinuses produce a gas called nitric oxide. When you breathe in through your nose, small amounts of this gas travel with the air into your lungs. Nitric oxide not only kills germs and viruses but also relaxes the muscles in the lungs with the result that the resistance in the airway decreases and the airflow to the lower lobs of the lungs where most of the gas exchange takes place increases. These effects help to lower your blood pressure and increase the oxygen-absorbing capacity of your lungs.
- Nose breathing helps to relax rigid muscles, and prevents other muscles from tightening. This leads to increased mobility throughout the body, which in turn helps to better oxygenate the muscles and reduces soreness after a workout.
- Optimal breathing is also important to maintain balance between oxygen and carbon dioxide in your blood. Mouth breathing lowers carbon dioxide levels fast. This may sound as a benefit but carbon dioxide is more than just a waste product as it plays an important role in how well your body can take up and use oxygen. Oxygen is carried around in the blood stream by red blood cells that contain the protein hemoglobin. Arriving at the tissues that need to be oxygenated, hemoglobin has to release the oxygen. The function of carbon dioxide is to enable hemoglobin

to release the oxygen to the tissues, a function that loses its effectiveness when not enough carbon dioxide is present.
- Mouth breathing can cause constriction of the carotid arteries. These arteries are located in the neck, one on each side. Their function is to supply blood to the brain, neck and face. The effect of mouth breathing is that it can reduce the supply of oxygen to the brain by half, which in turn often leads to feeling light headed. Even though it may feel like you're sucking in more oxygen when you breathe through your mouth, the opposite is in fact the case.

Nasal breathing has more benefits. Because of the resistance you experience with breathing through your nose due to the smaller passages of your nasal airways, you'll give your lungs a good workout which improves their flexibility.

Last but not least, nasal breathing is, due to decreased muscle and nerve tension throughout the body, associated with better posture and speech.

All of the benefits of nasal breathing listed above can only take place when you breathe through your nose and not through your mouth. The nose is a fundamental part of the respiratory system and should not be bypassed. Therefore the common recommendation; eat and speak through your mouth and breathe through your nose.

Many people deal with nasal congestion, which can make nasal breathing challenging. Light breathing helps to cope with this situation. It is also a good method to become used to breathing through your nose. Simply begin with taking small breaths in and out through your nose while sitting and at rest. When you feel comfortable, do the same during activities that are more physically demanding, and keep working your way up until you get used to breathing through your nose all the time.

It requires a few weeks to adjust to this new habit. Awareness is the key. Focus on your breathing and when you notice that you are breathing through your mouth, make no fuss of it, simply correct it and go back to nose breathing.

Staying On the Safe Side

Each of the five circles of safe and effective exercising are of equal importance as well as the sequence in which they appear.

The two first circles "Fundamental Laws of Strength Training" and "The Principles of Strength Training" form the foundation and preparation of circle three and four; "The Six-Step Effective Exercise Plan" and "The Full Body Workout."

When you create your own exercise program, go through the circles one to four to check for congruency. It can save you so much time and make your program so much more effective if you know what you're doing and make deliberate choices on the type of training program.

Although exercising can provide enormous health benefits both physically and mentally, if done in a manner that doesn't meet with the needs of your body and mind, you put yourself at risk for experiencing unwanted effects.

Be aware of your short- and long-term body responses that point toward these unwanted effects.

The most common example of a short-term body response after a workout is muscle soreness. There is nothing wrong with muscle soreness as long as it tapers off in two to three days. If it lasts longer, you very likely pushed yourself too much. Respect your body and learn from this lesson. Take a step back, let the soreness disappear and build-up more gradually when you pick up your workout routine.

Potentially more serious short-term body responses from exercising are acute injuries that present themselves with immediate pain, stiffness and spasms leading to immediate swelling, bruising, redness, tenderness and loss of normal function.

Minimizing the tissue damage and minimizing the inflammatory response are the two main goals to keep in mind. The best strategy for managing an acute injury is seeing a physician for a diagnosis as soon as possible, taking and keeping any load off the injured tissue, lying down to elevate and ice the injured tissue and applying a compression bandage.

Unwanted long-term body responses from exercising are overuse injuries. Examples are low-grade discomfort and stiffness in activities of daily living that don't disappear after a few days but keep lingering or even progress and lead to limping, swelling, tenderness to touch and loss of pain-free motion.

Instead of ignoring the discomfort or pain or taking painkillers, it is imperative to address the issue. Take rest, follow the strategy for acute injury and observe if the pain disappears or distinctly diminishes during 72 hours following onset of the discomfort or pain. A typical sign of overuse is pain within 2.5 centimetres of a joint or tendon or ligament attachment. Stay on the safe side and see a physician when the discomfort or pain persists.

Less known long-term body responses are those related to over training and can be both physical and mental.

Examples of physical responses are chronic tiredness, insomnia, loss of appetite, stomach discomfort and headaches.

Examples of mental responses include depression, apathy, low self-esteem, difficulty concentrating and sensitive to stress.

When you have pushed yourself to this level, the obvious recommendation can only be rest for a prolonged time. How long depends of course on the seriousness of the complaints. Listen to your body; it knows best.

Enjoy the Process

Although it is important to keep a good focus on your goals, it is also good to remember that, similar to what I wrote with regard to healthy nutrition, your body is not a machine and therefore won't always behave in accordance with what you think and plan.

Progress is never a linear process. Once you have begun your workout routine, it will take a number of weeks until your body gets the message and begins to improve and strengthen to withstand the repetitive challenges from the workouts.

Think of this, your body consists of eleven organ systems. Seven of them you see illustrated below. From left to right,

1. Skin
2. Respiratory system
3. Skeleton
4. Muscular system
5. Digestive system
6. Cardiopulmonary system
7. Nervous system

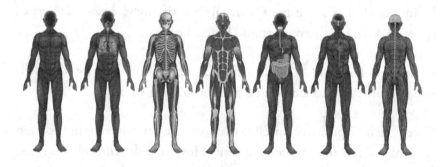

Body Organ Systems

The other 4 organ systems are:

8. Urinary system
9. Reproductive system
10. Hormonal/endocrine system
11. Lymphatic system

It is not realistic to expect that all those systems will improve their function linearly individually and collectively.

The sequence of body improvements when beginning a regular workout routine goes roughly as follows. First there is the learning curve for the brain that needs to figure out which muscle fibers to fire and when. Chances are that you will feel a bit awkward when doing the exercises for the first time. Please give your brain and your entire nervous system a bit of time. It will soon go better.

After the first neurological improvements, tendons and ligaments begin to strengthen, facilitating a movement through the full range of motion. Once these are on their way with improving their function, the muscles will follow with growing in strength and size.

It will take 5 to 6 weeks to reach this point. From there you can expect a gradual improvement in all other body functions. It only makes sense that this whole process takes time. Some body functions will improve faster and pull others forward, whereas other body functions stay a bit behind because they simply need more time.

There is no strict schedule. Each body is unique and enters the stage with a background and level of health and fitness that is different from any other person.

Because you will spend most of the time in the process of working toward your goals, you might as well enjoy it. When you re-establish the relationship with your body and mind, you will learn things you wish you had been aware of earlier in your life. It really will be a wonderful experience. The outcome you may expect is that your body will reward you with enhanced quality of life every week you follow through with your workout routine.

The Fifth Circle of Safe and Effective Exercising, "Mastering Your Exercise Habits"

Let's see where we are now and do a quick recap again.

In Part One we covered some basics about the nervous system, in particular the brain. How it processes the signals coming from our five senses and how the various parts of the brain play a role in the forming of beliefs, habits and expectations that ultimately shape the person we are, our personality, our self-image.

The Two-Step technique of prolonged pointed attention with vivid creative imagination provided the method to first replace negative thoughts to improve overall well-being and through this health and performance and second to consistently work on improving our self-image; how we perceive ourselves.

In Part Two went over the four circles of healthy nutrition, "Quality", "Quantity", "Timing" and "Balance", seen from the body's perspective, meaning that we looked at the nutrients the body thrives instead of what we would like it to thrive on. Part Two closed with "Mastering Your Eating Habits" in which we discussed setting goals, mastering stress, applying the Two-Step technique and the routine of Focus – Action – Reflection, geared to healthy nutrition, how to stay motivated and the role of willpower.

In this final part we'll bring it all together, building upon your self-image, establishing supportive eating habits and creating a regular workout routine, all three with the one aim to enjoy the benefits of a healthy lifestyle and improved quality of life.

Making Safe and Effective Exercising Part of Your Healthy Life Style

Creating a regular workout routine is what many people find the most challenging aspect of maintaining a healthy lifestyle. Point is that whatever the nature of these challenges, they are much easier to deal with if you know which buttons to push.

The buttons I refer to are the feel-good neurotransmitters I mentioned in Part One; serotonin, dopamine, endorphins, anandamide and GABA. Elevated levels of these neurotransmitters simply make it impossible to feel sad, depressed and stressed.

Regular exercising is a proven method to increase the levels of these feel-good neurotransmitters. Aside from health effects that occur over time such as losing weight and improving strength, stamina and flexibility, regular exercising also provides instant gratification in the form of feeling relaxed, happy and in control.

Moreover, feeling relaxed and happy means that the parasympathetic nervous system dominates and metabolic processes such as digestion, assimilation, healing and recovery can take place without interruption.

Safe and effective exercising is nothing less than a life elixir that instantaneously improves quality of life.

Even though your reasoning and logical thinking conscious mind may understand the benefits of regular exercising, your emotional subconscious mind may hold different beliefs. As always, it likes to hold on to what it sees as known and familiar and therefore as true and safe. If a sedentary lifestyle and 60 pounds of excess body weight fits with what it sees as known and familiar, then that is what it likes to hold on to even though it doesn't serve the needs of your body and your goals in life.

Understanding this characteristic, you know that you will have to speak the subconscious mind's language to make it accept the new habits as the new standard to hold on to, meaning that you will have to apply gentle persistence to instill the new habits into your subconscious mind.

Crucial element in this learning process is avoiding any type of stress, as this will immediately put an end to the process, no matter how hard the conscious mind will attack and punish the subconscious mind for its disobedience.

Applying gentle persistence begins with consciously thinking throughout the day for a few days about the exercise routine you want to establish. The technique of prolonged pointed attention to fill your mind with positive thoughts about the benefits of regular exercising, especially those that give instant gratification, is the obvious first step to prepare the subconscious mind for step two, the technique of vivid creative imagination.

The purpose is to ease your subconscious mind into the idea of installing and maintaining the new habit of regular exercising. Be persistent in feeding your subconscious mind with positive thoughts about exercising but don't rush it. In other words, use your willpower wisely. This is an indispensable part of the process. Don't skip it, enjoy it.

This preparation phase of step one is a perfect moment to think of a place for working out, in a gym or at home, equipment, comfortable clothing, pen and paper to keep track of your results and other things you may need.

Then it is time for step two, applying the technique of vivid creative imagination, following the same format to install healthy nutrition habits.

Picture that big white screen again in front of you and project yourself onto the screen going through a normal day before implementing the new habit of regular exercising. Let this picture then disappear to the right, representing the past, and move in from the left side of the screen, representing the present, a picture of you performing the new habits as if they already were part of your everyday life.

Do this as vividly and as detailed as possible to promote the release of the feel-good neurotransmitters, your big allies that support you in the process. To enhance the experience, go into the screen and into yourself and look out of the eyes while you are performing the actions.

Remember using your senses. Look very carefully at all the details. Begin with seeing yourself reviewing the "Time-Bender" exercise, and preparing your workout sheet. Be aware of the day of the week and your environment. Hear supportive comments from people. Add colors, smells, sounds of music and so on.

See through your eyes when you are preparing yourself for your workout. Notice the clothes and shoes you are wearing, the weights you are holding in your hands, if any, and the towel and water bottle you have with you.

Keep looking through your eyes when you are doing the exercises. Feel your feet pressing against the floor, how you work through the full range of motion, the contracting and stretching of your muscles, and focus on your technique and breathing.

When you have completed the workout, notice what you see during the cooldown, hear what you say to yourself and hear from others, feel the warmth of your body, the beating of your heart, and realize how energized and full of confidence you feel.

Focus on and analyze carefully the healthy food items you eat after a workout. When you feel, smell, taste and chew your food slowly, look inside yourself and follow the food from your mouth to your stomach into your intestines where the nutrients are absorbed and transported to your organs and recovering muscles. Notice how your body as a whole benefits from eating healthy food, how it re-energizes you and makes you stronger.

Making the entire experience as real and vivid as you can and as if already a reality is essential to ingrain the routine and associated brain pattern as quickly as possible. The more you mix the experience with emotion, the more feel-good neurotransmitters will be released that help with this process.

When you're finished with that days' practice, go back to step one to hold on to the good feelings and intentions, act upon them and create an ongoing cycle of step one and step two, day after day.

Similar to Part One and Two, using affirmations are another way to reach your subconscious mind in order to install habits that support your intentions of living a healthy lifestyle. The affirmations below combine building self-image and healthy eating habits with the habit of safe and effective exercising.

"I feel confident, happy and safe because I see myself becoming stronger and losing weight. I am organizing my days using the "Time-Bender" exercise, work out twice a week, eat healthy, get enough rest and sleep and keep my body and mind relaxed at all times. I am aware that because I structure my days, I feel more relaxed and in control of my thoughts and behavior. I know with certainty that these components of my exercise and nutrition program make me feel and look strong, energetic and confident and allow me to perform at my best. This is my life and this is how I want to live."

"I am planning my days, work out two times per week, eat healthy food, fill my mind with happy and supportive thoughts and give my body enough rest and sleep for healing and recovery. I realize that these healthy lifestyle habits support my intentions to live a healthy, fulfilling and purposeful life."

"I feel better every day and fully enjoy creating the life I choose to live."

Use the Step-Two vivid creative imagination practice and the affirmations as concepts to adjust to your own situation. The variations can of course be endless.

Remember to keep these rules in mind,

Stay in the present, as if the desired outcome is already a fact. Do not say things like "I'm going to" or "Next time I will". Those words point at a desired outcome in the future.

Avoid negatives because they unconsciously set you up for failure and frustration. Examples are cannot, try, could have, but, might, should, would have, must, maybe, couldn't, some day.

Record the script and listen to it 3 to 4 times. Although you may find listening to your own voice a bit awkward, don't let these emotions get between you and your goals. The pay-off is two-fold. First, your brain can concentrate on one thing which is listening and second, the fact that you are listening to your own voice makes the affirmation much more effective.

Hold on to your Anchors and the routine of Focus – Action – Reflection

With so much going on in body and mind when implementing all the action steps related to healthy nutrition, and safe and effective exercising, it can be helpful to hold on to a number of anchors to keep yourself on track toward a healthy lifestyle.

Luckily, you have a good number that give you the certainty and peace of mind you need to enjoy every hour of the process. Here they are:

1. Time-Bender
2. The Weekly Meal Plan with Shopping List
3. Food and Fluid Journal
4. Template Shopping List
5. The Healthy Nutrition Plan
6. Checklist Achieving and Maintaining a Healthy Weight
7. The Six-Step Healthy Exercise Plan
8. Checklist Optimizing Results Training Program
9. Workout Journal
10. Your Two-Step technique of Prolonged Pointed Attention combined with Vivid Creative Imagination
11. The affirmations
12. Your Lifestyle Change Goal-Setting Plan and Journal
13. A support system
14. A reward system

Review these anchors and make from "Focus – Action – Reflection" an ongoing routine. Again, enjoy the process. Be the observer, the witness of the responses of your body and mind, notice how the two interact, stay in your role of conductor and make adjustments when and where necessary.

Once More Part One
"Mastering Your Life"

It is here that we connect back to "Mastering Your Life" to further embed "Eating for Life" and "Moving for Life". At this stage, you may have drawn the conclusion that the two easiest to tackle components of living a healthy lifestyle are in fact healthy nutrition and safe and effective exercising. You are right about your conclusion.

The problem is not in these two components, although most people think it is, hence the recommendation move more, eat less and just do it. Problem solved.

The real problem is mastering the numerous intangible processes that take place in our brain and can turn our life into heaven or hell.

The tool we can rely on to master these processes is our conscious mind, home of our willpower. The good thing is that we all have the ability to develop and train our conscious mind, meaning that we all have the ability to bring our actions in alignment with our intentions and move our life in the direction we want it to go.

Nothing worthwhile ever comes easy. It requires effort but as long as you embrace the process, see obstacles as your opportunity for growth and keep working with gentle persistence, you'll inevitably get better every week at mastering the automatic reactions from the subconscious mind.

The following chapter may give you some valuable tips to help you with further strengthening your willpower, crown jewel of the conscious mind.

Nine Ways To Build Your Willpower

Willpower enters the stage again in this chapter. What we covered in the previous chapters about willpower is that it lives in our conscious mind and that, when used wisely, it is the single most important tool to manage our thoughts, feelings, behavior and change our habits to make them consistent with our intentions in life.

One may argue that talent, good looks and charisma play important key roles in life as well, but since neither of them can exist without the drive, control and direction coming from willpower, it is the latter that eventually outperforms all three.

This chapter is about how to improve the function of this crown jewel of the conscious mind. Reality shows that those who know how to master their responses and actions best are the ones who are the most flexible in their behavior and the most successful in every aspect of life.

They are in general healthier and happier, make more money, enjoy fulfilling and lasting relationships, are better at handling stress, conflicts and setbacks, experience more job satisfaction and feel often inspired and supported by something bigger outside of them.

Willpower is in all of us, but as with so many things in life, if we don't constantly cultivate and nourish it, it will deteriorate and never grow to its full potential, putting us at risk for living an unsatisfying life without direction or purpose.

Whether you want to build upon your self-image, improve your eating habits, hold on to a regular workout routine or wish to get more pleasure out of any other aspect of life, willpower is your friend and ally. Aside from the 14 anchors mentioned above, you'll find below a list with suggestions that build upon the anchors and offer additional insights to make your willpower and eventually your life flourish.

1. Healthy eating habits are of course at the top of the list. Extensively covered in this book it is the first way to help your willpower. First and for all, healthy food keeps your microbiome happy. Aside of the many other tasks they take care of, they produce 80 to 90 percent of the feel-good neurotransmitter serotonin, keep the intestinal lining healthy to prevent invaders from entering the blood stream, and stimulate the millions of nerve cells that make up the vagus nerve, which connects the gut-brain with the head-brain.

   Although glucose is the main source of energy for muscles and brain, you want to avoid food that spikes the glucose levels in your blood since it impairs about every body function, mentally as well as physically. Vegetables and moderate amounts of healthy fats and plant-based protein will keep your blood sugar levels stable and your body and mind function at their best.

2. Safe and effective exercising is the next sure way to improve brain-health and willpower. Feeling stressed, sad, depressed and anxious are devastating for willpower and numerous studies have learned that regular exercising helps to alleviate these conditions. Exercise also helps to normalize blood sugar levels, which in turn helps with preventing nervousness, over-activity and varying energy levels.

   Lastly, exercising stimulates the production of new brain cells or grey matter and myelin, the whitish insulation wrapped around the axons of many nerve fibers, increasing the speed at which impulses move. The prefrontal cortex, home of the conscious mind and willpower, in particular benefits from exercising.

3. Meditation is another proven way to boost brain function and willpower. Meditation helps with centering your attention, controlling impulses, improving awareness and stress management. Scientists noticed physical changes in brain structure in the form of new brain tissue and increased neural connections due to an increased blood flow to the prefrontal cortex. Your brain adapts to meditation in the same way your muscles adapt to strength training. Even if it is only one minute you can meditate, never skip a day.

4. Slow and deep breathing from your belly promotes relaxation as discussed in Parts One and Two. The conscious mind including willpower can only function optimally when we feel relaxed. Stress-reactions from the amygdala immediately diminish the function of the conscious mind, which in turn impairs clear thinking and self-control. Exhaling a few seconds longer than inhaling is a first simple step to reduce feelings of stress.

5. Sufficient sleep and rest are essential for optimal performance during the day. Lack of sleep raises the risk for accidents, depression and a number of other health issues. 7 to 8 hours of sleep per night is what we need to keep our body and brain healthy. With regard to brain health, it is good to know that our glymphatic system, which is our brain's waste removal system, is only active during deep sleep.

6. Focus on improving your self-image. A sound and solid self-image has a great positive impact on brain health and willpower. It is the main message of Part One of this book. A healthy and strong self-image is a first condition to reflect diligently, patiently and consistently upon your thoughts, feelings, beliefs, habits and expectations and decide which aren't consistent with your goals in life and need to be replaced.

7. Make an inventory of the challenges and set-backs you can expect, think of ways to deal with them and see them as opportunities for growth. This attitude helps you to keep your mind relaxed and makes it easier to overcome the obstacles.

Wherever you see people succeed, it is always by accepting and expecting temporary defeats. Turning temporary defeats into permanent defeats is a choice and the consequence of an unhealthy self-image and attitude.

This may sound a bit harsh but sudden automatic success seldom sustains. Think of the rise and fall people often go through after winning a lottery or inheriting an important position.

Too many children and people grow up and live in a protected world where challenges are taken away from them and every difficulty in their life is smoothened with quick fixes. Comforted, pampered and rewarded for every achievement, they never get the opportunity to build the mental strength to face and handle the challenges that eventually and inevitably will come on their path. The moment life puts them to the test, they stand empty handed and see no other solutions than to quickly give up, reach out for quick fixes or rely on the help of others.

8. Keep a journal. It is a fact that people who write down their goals, describe their successes and challenges and work out strategies to follow the process and their progress are more successful. Keeping a journal helps you to organize your thoughts and supports clear thinking for successfully applying the routine of Focus – Action – Reflection. It motivates, holds you accountable and cultivates the positive willpower necessary to pursue.

What derives from keeping a journal is a master-student frame of mind. A master keeps an eye on the bigger picture, knows that learning can only happen in a safe environment and that patience and gentle persistence are essential to keep moving forward.

It is for this purpose that you'll find in this book a "Lifestyle Change Goal-Setting Plan and Journal".

9. As simple as it sounds, the effects a neat and clean house and workplace have on peace of mind and therefore willpower can be profound. Getting rid of chaos and clutter, and organizing your environment does the same thing for your mind.

It is one of the easiest ways to put an end to those time consuming, annoying and energy draining activities of trying to find back lost items and so on.

A very welcome other side effect of a neat and clean environment is the elimination of distractions. A mind at ease helps to control behavior and limits unnecessary actions. As a result it will be easier to remain focused and center your willpower.

What the previous nine points have in common is that they create structure, keep you away from stress and put you in charge of your life.

Whatever the nature of your thoughts and feelings, the single most important action of your conscious mind is to move and keep your thoughts and feelings away from the amygdala's panic-button.

Without exception, every time an experience we go through pushes that button, stress-reactions begin to occur. They may not always be distinctly visible but they are always there and will always affect our mental and physical processes. The harder the panic-button gets hit, the less control the conscious mind can carry out to the point that it becomes fully overruled.

Learning to identify the symptoms of stress in your life and remaining aware of where you are every moment of the day opens the door to fully exercise the qualities of the conscious mind including self-control and willpower, enabling you to be the creator of your life instead of being the mindless absorber that takes in and acts upon whatever comes to you through your senses.

How To Go From Here

The aim of this book is to provide you with a flight plan and runway that enables you to take off toward a healthier and therefore more fulfilling and rewarding life. I hope that this book has given you insights about the body mind and that you, as the true expert of your own body and mind, have begun to explore your feelings and thoughts that have resulted in the beliefs, expectations and habits that created your life.

Although healthy nutrition and safe and effective exercising form the core of this book, they make up only one piece of the wellness wheel. Since everything in life is connected and the tools and techniques described in this book can easily be modified and applied to the other five aspects of the wellness wheel, I encourage you to find out if you can, if you haven't already decided to do so.

Is this the time and place to say goodbye and wish you all the best? Not necessarily. Feel free to visit my website www.masteringwillpower.com for more information or to leave your questions.

If there is one thing that stands out in this book, it is that you can change your life.

Dive in, get what is yours and have the time of your life.

Patrick Streppel.

About The Author

Patrick's aim has always been to create positive changes in his life and that of others that go beyond mediocrity. Whether it was during the nearly ten months of his travels with his wife Denise on bicycles through parts of Southeast Asia and Europe, as real-estate broker in Amsterdam or as owner and manager of a tourist business elsewhere in The Netherlands, Patrick's aim has always been to go the extra mile for others and himself.

Taking new pathways means choosing for experiences and challenges that are often unpredictable. Most of them are good and even beautiful, whereas others turn out to be serious obstacles. They are all part of the game. What they have in common is that they shape you into the person you need to become to realize your dreams.

The dream in Southeast Asia was to complete the journey, meet with wonderful people and see all the special places despite the problems related to travel conditions, equipment, eating and drinking, shelter for the night, health and weather.

The dream in Amsterdam, after obtaining real-estate broker credentials and moving up from employee to employer, was building a respected and thriving real estate business. The challenge that arose after realizing that dream was accepting that it was time to move on and leave a well-established and well-paying business behind.

The next dream emerged in a rural area north of Amsterdam where Patrick and his wife Denise spent ten years on renovating an old farmhouse into a charming family home with attached comfortable hotel for 34 guests.

Patrick currently lives with his family of five in Ontario, Canada where he founded and operates since 2010 a small personal fitness training business.

People have always been the binding element in the dreams, successes and challenges during the past thirty years.

Regardless of how big or small a dream, not one can be achieved without being confronted with obstacles. Maintaining a positive and persistent mindset forms the key in overcoming challenges of any kind. You can deal with them, you always can. Problems and obstacles can only exist by the mercy of not having found the solution yet, which could be waiting just around the corner.

A positive and persistent mindset includes choosing to feel strong, happy, kind, grateful and resourceful no matter what. The law of the Universe says that there is no receiving without giving first. The magical words that open all doors are how can I help? The magical words that will then soon come your way are how can I help you?

People may often be part of a problem, they are always part of the solution. Help them, go beyond their expectations and they will help you beyond your expectations.

Vivid creative imagination that perceives a desired outcome as if already reality pulled Patrick and Denise through when pursuing dreams and dealing with challenges that could sometimes be severe, as was the case when they had to fear for the life of their newborn son while being in the midst of renovating the farmhouse and building the hotel business.

The positive and persistent mindset that brought him to where he is now in life remains at the core of his role as husband, father, business owner, personal fitness trainer and nutrition and life coach.

His current professional services focus on helping men and women after forty optimizing their health with customized programs comprising healthy nutrition, safe and effecting exercising and establishing habits that support a healthy lifestyle they can maintain for life.

Additional Resources

Author	Book Title	ISBN
Baechle, Thomas R. and Westcott, Wayne L.	Strength Training for Older Adults	978-0-7360-7581-7
Bompa, Tudor O. PhD and Carrera, Michalel C.	Periodization Training for Sports	978-0-7360-5559-8
Campbell, Colin T., PhD and Campbell II, Thomas M., MD	The China Study	978-193210066-2
David, Marc	Nourishing Wisdom	978-0-517-88129-3
David, Marc	Slow Down Diet	978-159477060-9
Davis, William, MD	Wheat Belly	978-1-44341-273-5
Mercola, Joseph, Dr	Effortless, Healing	978-0-553-41797-5
McGuff, Doug, MD and Little, John	Body by Science	978-0-07-159717-3
Moss, Michael	Salt, Sugar, Fat	978-0-7710-5710-6
Perlmutter, David, MD	Brain Maker	978-0-316-38010-2
Ready, Romilla and Burton, Kate	Neuro-linguistic Programming for Dummies	978-1-119-10611-1
Salatin, Joel	Folks, this ain't normal	978-0-89296-820-6
Taubes, Gary	Why we get fat	978-0-307-27270-6
	Foundations of Professional Personal Training	978-0-7360-6910-6

"Brain & Body Fit After Forty"
"Time Bender Exercise"

| _____ Day | Time | |
Type of Activity: (sleep, work, break, eating, relax, other)	Start	End

Brain & Body
Fit
After Forty

7 Days Mealplan

Meal Suggestions For An Entire Week From Breakfast
to Dinner and Snacks With Shopping List

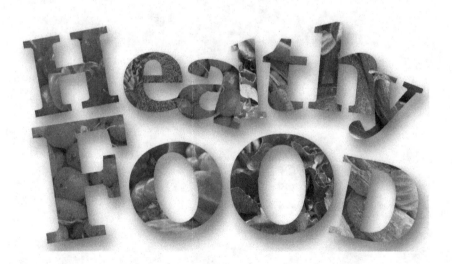

Table of Contents

Day 1

Breakfast

Yoghurt with nuts and fruit

Prep time 10 min

Ingredients:

1 cup plain (Greek) yoghurt

½ cup fresh/frozen berries

½ cup raw walnuts/almonds/pecans

Process:

Mix all ingredients together and enjoy!

Snack

1 organic Apple

Lunch

Chicken Salad

Prep time 15 min, cook time 15 min.

Ingredients:

- 1/2 chicken breasts, sliced
- 1 celery stalk, chopped
- 1/4 cucumber, chopped

- ½ red onion, thinly sliced
- 1 tomato cubed or 1/3 cup cherry tomatoes
- 1/3 cup olives (optional)
- 1-2 cups spring salad greens or romaine heart and/or baby spinach
- ¼ cup broccoli, chopped
- Dressing: balsamic vinaigrette= 3 tbsp balsamic vinegar
- 2 cloves garlic(minced)
- ¼ cup red onion(diced)
- 1 tbsp Dijon mustard
- ½ tsp each salt and pepper
- 1cup extra virgin olive oil
- Mix all ingredients and toss with salad

Process:

- Preheat grill to medium-high heat or cook in a skillet
- Grill chicken breasts for 7-10 min. per side, flipping once.
- Slice chicken into ¼-inch stripes.
- Rinse and chop all vegetables, toss them with spring salad greens.

Top with grilled chicken, drizzle with dressing and serve.

Snack

2 stalk organic celery and some cherry tomatoes

Dinner

Asian Stir-fry Beef Broccoli

Prep time 10 min, cook time 10 min.

Ingredients:

- 1 tbsp butter or coconut oil
- 2 cloves garlic, minced
- 1 tbsp ginger, minced
- 100 gram (3-4 oz) beef for stir fry, cut into slices
- 1-2 cup of broccoli in pieces chopped
- ¼ cup (green) onion, thinly sliced
- 2 tbs coconut aminos (=soy-free seasoning sauce made from coconut tree sap) or organic soy sauce
- Salt and pepper to taste
- 1 tbs Thai fish sauce
- ½ tsp red pepper flakes
- 1 tbs sesame seed

Process:

- Heat butter/coconut oil in a wok
- Add garlic and ginger, sauté for 2 minutes
- Add steak, stirring frequently until fully browned
- Add broccoli, continue to sauté over high heat
- Add green onion and 1 tbsp of oil if necessary
- Poor in coconut aminos or soy sauce and season with salt, pepper and red pepper flakes and fish sauce
- Continue to sauté for another 2-3 minutes
- Garnish with a sprinkle of sesame seeds and serve

Desert/Snack

1/3 cup plain (Greek and/or 3 %) yogurt with ¼ cup (blue)berries.

Day 2

Breakfast

Yoghurt with nuts and fruit

Prep time 10 min, cook time 10 min.

Ingredients:

- 1 cup plain (Greek) yoghurt
- ½ cup fresh/frozen berries
- ½ cup raw walnuts/almonds/pecans

Process:

Mix all ingredients together and enjoy!

Snack

10 walnuts and 10 raw almonds

Lunch

Scrambled eggs with salmon

Prep time 10 min, cook time 10 min.

Ingredients:

- 1 tsp coconut oil/butter
- ¼ cup (red) onion, chopped
- 2 eggs
- 2 oz smoked wild salmon, chopped

- 1 big tomato, sliced
- 1 tsp capers
- 1 tsp chopped parsley
- Pepper to taste

Process:

- Heat coconut oil/butter in skillet
- Sauté onion
- Whisk 2 eggs in bowl
- Mix chopped salmon with the eggs
- Pour eggs and salmon over the onions
- Cook, stirring gently to scramble
- Serve over sliced tomato and garnish with capers, parsley and pepper

Snack/Desert

Orange

Diner

Zucchini lasagne (serves 2, so keep ½ as leftover)

Prep time 15 min, cook time 25 min.

Ingredients:

- 150 gram ground beef
- 2 cloves garlic, minced
- 1 onion, chopped
- 1 small green pepper, chopped
- 1 small can tomato paste
- 15 oz tomato sauce

- 1 tbsp fresh parsley
- 1 tbsp basil
- 1 tbsp oregano
- Salt and pepper to taste
- 1 zucchini, sliced thinly
- 1 ¼ cups mushrooms, sliced
- Fresh grated cheese (about 1 cup)

Process:

- Brown the ground beef in a large skillet
- Add garlic, onion and green pepper
- Stir in tomato paste and tomato sauce
- Add in parsley, basil, oregano, salt and pepper
- Bring sauce to a light boil, then remove from heat
- Grease a 9" x 13" baking dish with coconut oil/butter
- Place a thin layer (1/2 inch) of the sauce in the dish
- Layer zucchini and mushroom over sauce, and repeat, alternating layering of sauce in the dish
- Bake lasagne at 325 Fahrenheit for 15 minutes, covered with foil
- After 15 minutes, remove foil, add cheese increase temperature to 350 Fahrenheit and bake for an additional 10 minutes.

Snack/Dessert

Baked apple/nut crisp (serves 2, so keep ½ for later this week)

Prep time 15 min, cook time 45 min.

Ingredients:

- 2 apples, peeled cored and diced
- 1 Tbsp. butter
- 1/3 cup apple cider (no sugar added)
- ½ Tbsp. maple syrup

- ½ Tbsp. cinnamon
- ½ tsp. nutmeg
- 1/2 tsp. cardamom (optional)
- 1/4 cup almonds
- 1/4 cup walnuts
- 1/4 cup pecans
- 1/2 cup almond flour
- 2 tbs unsweetened shredded coconut
- 1 Tbsp. maple syrup
- 2 tbs melted coconut oil/butter
- ½ tsp. cinnamon

Process:

- Preheat oven to 350°F.
- In a small saucepan over medium-high heat, melt the butter, then add the cider, maple syrup, and spices.
- Whisk together and bring to a gentle boil.
- Let boil for about 10-15 minutes to reduce and thicken.
- Meanwhile, put diced apples in a heatproof bowl.
- When cider mixture is ready, pour over apples and toss to coat.
- Pour apples into baking dish.
- In a medium bowl, stir together all the topping ingredients and then spread evenly over the apples in the baking dish.
- Cover dish with tin foil and place in the oven, setting timer for 45 minutes.
- When the timer goes off, remove foil and bake for another 10 minutes to brown the topping.
- Remove from oven, let cool for a few minutes, then serve it up with a shovel.

Day 3

Breakfast

Oates Pancake with Apples (see recipe day 7 is enough for 2 breakfast servings)

Snack

1 cup of raw veggies

Lunch

Mixed Salad with leftover smoked salmon

Prep time 10 min

Ingredients:

- ½ cup cucumber
- ½ cups grape tomatoes
- 1 cup baby spinach
- ¼ cup olives
- ½ tsp basil,
- ½ tsp oregano
- 1 clove garlic, minced
- 2 tbsp extra-virgin olive oil
- 1 tbsp balsamic vinegar
- Leftover smoked salmon
- Cracked black pepper/salt/mustard to taste

Process:

- Rinse and peel cucumber and chop into bite sized pieces
- Rinse grape tomatoes and slice in half
- Thinly slice basil, chop oregano, mince garlic
- Toss all ingredients with the olives, baby spinach and salmon in a medium bowl, drizzle with olive oil and balsamic vinegar and sprinkle with black pepper.

Snack

1 Orange or Tangerine

Dinner

Baked chicken thighs with veggies

Prep time 5 min, cook time 30 min.

Ingredients:

- 2 bone-in, skin on chicken thighs (preferably organic or antibiotic/hormone free!)
- 1 tbs butter/coconut oil
- 1 shallot, minced
- 2 garlic cloves – minced
- Salt and pepper to taste

Veggies (to your own taste). You probably have bell pepper, onion and broccoli left, so make an easy going stir-fry dish and add some Thai fish sauce, red pepper flakes to taste.

Process:

- Heat butter/coconut oil and bake thighs in skillet.
- Add shallots and garlic, sprinkle the skin with pepper/salt.
- Bake 25-30 min or until juices run clear.

Desert/Snack

1/3 cup cottage cheese or plain yoghurt with fresh/frozen berries

Day 4

Breakfast

Egg Muffins (6-8 muffins so more than enough for 2x breakfast, you can freeze leftovers)

Prep time 10-15 min, cook time 20 min.

Ingredients:

- ½ tsp coconut oil/butter
- ½ medium onion, chopped
- 1 cup broccoli, chopped
- ¼ green pepper, chopped
- ¼ red pepper, chopped
- 6 eggs
- Salt and pepper to taste

Process:

- Preheat oven to 400 Fahrenheit
- Grease muffin tin with coconut oil/butter
- Rinse and chop all vegetables into ¼ inch pieces

- Divide vegetables evenly between muffin tins
- Whisk the eggs, pour into the tins, dividing evenly
- Sprinkle with salt and pepper, then stir the vegetable and egg mixture briefly
- Bake the egg muffins in the oven for 18 – 20 minutes

Snack

1 serving of fresh fruit

Lunch

Tuna-Avocado Salad

Ingredients:

- 2 cups mixed greens or baby spinach
- ½ carrot, shredded
- 2 ounces tuna (1 small can)
- 1 tbsp parsley
- 1 avocado, cubed
- 2 lime wedges

Process:

- Combine the greens and carrot in a bowl
- Add tuna and cilantro and toss to combine
- Add the avocado and squeeze the lime wedges just before serving
- Toss and serve immediately
- Add olive oil/vinegar dressing as made before

Dinner

Leftover Zuchini Lasagne

Desert/Snack

Leftover Apple-Crisp

Day 5

Breakfast

Egg Muffins from yesterday

Snack

1 organic banana

Lunch

Greek Salad

Prep time 10 min

Ingredients:

- 2 cups spring mixed greens
- 1 tomato chopped
- ½ green bell pepper, thinly sliced
- ½ red onion, thinly sliced
- ¼ cup capers
- ¼ cup olives
- ½ cup feta cheese crumbled

Dressing:

- juice of 1 lemon
- ¼ cup extra virgin olive oil
- 1 glove garlic (minced)
- 1 tsp dried oregano
- salt and pepper to taste
- Squeeze lemon juice into a small mixing bowl
- whisk in olive oil, garlic, oregano
- add salt and pepper and toss with salad

Process:

- Toss spring greens with tomatoes, green bell pepper, feta, red onion and sliced cucumber in a bowl
- Top salad with capers and olives
- Add dressing.

Snack

Orange or Organic Apple

Diner

Beef Burrito/Omelet, prep time 10 min, cook time 15 min.

Ingredients:

- 100 gram ground beef
- 1 tbs butter
- 2 eggs
- 1 tbs butter/ coconut oil
- 1/4 cup red onion, thinly sliced
- 1 cup spring greens

- 1/3 cucumber
- 1 tomato
- ½ green bell pepper
- Cilantro/parsley for garnish

Seasoning:

- 1tsp cumin
- 1 tsp onion powder
- tsp garlic powder
- 1 tsp paprika
- salt and pepper to taste

Process:

- Whisk eggs and set aside
- Heat butter in a skillet and brown the beef while stirring, add onion and spices
- In another skillet cook the omelet and after flipping over, add the beef on top and fold the omelet
- Toss spring greens with tomatoes, green bell pepper, red onion and sliced cucumber in a bowl
- Top salad with capers and olives
- Add dressing and serve as side dish with the beef burrito/omelet

Snack

2 squares of extra dark (at least 70% cocoa) chocolate.

Day 6

Breakfast

Smoothie with Avocado & Spinach

Prep time 10 min

Ingredients:

- 1 cup plain (Greek) yoghurt
- 1 banana
- 2 tbsp ground flaxseed
- ½ avocado
- 1 handful baby spinach
- about ½ cup water with fresh squeezed lemon juice of ½ lemon

Process:

Put all ingredients in a blender and blend until smooth. Add more water if too thick.

Snack

1 organic banana

Lunch

Mixed salad with avocado & cheese

Prep time 10 min, cook time 10 min.

Ingredients:

- Mix green salad (2 cups) with the other ½ avocado chopped and 2 slices of cheese cut in pieces.
- Add a variety of colored veggies (about 1 cup) as you have in stock in the fridge.
- Dressing from olive oil, balsamic vinegar, pepper, salt and mustard to taste.

Snack

1/3 cup of raw walnuts and almonds

Dinner

Quinoa-Stuffed Bell Peppers (2 servings, so you can have 1 for lunch another day)

Prep time 20 min, cook time 30 min.

Ingredients:

- ¼ cup almonds slivered
- ½ cup quinoa (cooked as described on package)
- 2 bell peppers
- 1 tbsp butter
- 1 onion chopped
- 1 glove garlic chopped
- 1/2 package (10 ounce) fresh spinach
- ¼ cup feta cheese crumbled
- 1 small can tomato paste
- 1 tomato
- ½ tsp Italian seasoning
- optional: small bowl of salad (made from what is left in your fridge).

Process:

- Cook (roast) the almonds in a small skillet, medium heat, stirring often till light brown and set aside.
- cook the quinoa as described on the package.
- Bring a large pot of water to a boil.
- Cut off and reserve the tops of the bell peppers and remove the seeds and ribs.
- Add the peppers to the boiling water and cook for 3 minutes. Drain.
- in the same pot heat the butter and cook the onion, garlic for 5 minutes, add the spinach and cook for 2 minutes.
- Remove the pot from the heat and add feta, almonds, quinoa to the spinach mixture.
- Arrange the peppers in a shallow baking dish, cover loosely with foil and cook for about 30 min in over at 350 degrees F.
- Meanwhile, in a saucepan add tomato paste, Italian seasoning and chopped tomato with 1/3 cup water, heat and stir. Poor sauce over the stuffed bell peppers and enjoy!
- Optional; serve with a small bowl of salad, made from "what is in the fridge left at the end of your week" like lettuce, veggies and drizzle with olive oil, balsamic vinegar, pepper and salt.

Snack

1/3 cup cottage cheese or plain yoghurt with fresh/frozen berries

Day 7

Breakfast

Oatmeal Pancakes with Apples (enough for 2x breakfast, see day 3)

Prep time 10 min, cook time 15 min.

Ingredients:

- ¾ cup buttermilk
- 1/3 cup whole wheat flour
- 1/3 cup instant rolled oats
- 1 tbs buttermilk
- 1 tbs melted butter
- 1 tsp baking powder
- ¼ tsp baking soda
- Pinch of cinnamon and ½ tsp for the apples1 organic apple peeled and chopped
- Pinch of nutmeg
- Butter to cook pancakes

Process:

- In a large bowl combine buttermilk, oats, flour milk, melted butter, baking powder and soda, cinnamon and nutmeg.
- Stir gently to combine.
- Set the batter aside for a few minutes
- Combine the apple, cinnamon and stir it in the batter till well mixed.
- Heat 1 tbsp butter in a large skillet and scoop ¼ cup portions of batter into the skillet.
- Cook for 2-3 minutes or until small bubbles form in the top of the batter.
- Flip over and cook for another 2 minutes.

Snack

A handful of raw veggies

Lunch

1 Stuffed bell pepper left over from yesterday

Snack

1 banana

Dinner

Stir It Up Chicken and snow peas

Prep time 15 min, cook time 10 min.

Ingredients:

- 1 tbs butter/coconut oil
- ¼ tsp red pepper flakes
- 1 small chicken breast in pieces
- ½ cup frozen/fresh snow peas
- 1/3 cup sliced carrots
- 1 medium onion, chopped
- 2 gloves garlic minced
- ½ cup sliced bell pepper
- 2 tbs almonds
- 1 tbs organic soy sauce
- Thai fish sauce to taste
- Brown rice cooked

Process:

- Heat the oil at medium heat and add the onion, chicken, garlic and stir fry for 3 minutes.
- Add all the veggies and cook for another 3 minutes, stirring often.
- Add fish sauce and soy sauce to taste.
- Serve over the rice

Snack

2 pieces of extra dark chocolate

Grocery List for 7 days meal plan (1 person)

- 10 (organic) eggs
- 2 small chicken breast (or 1 big one)
- 1 Romaine heart
- 1 box mixed (spring) greens
- 1 box baby spinach
- 1 small can tuna
- 2 can tomato paste
- 100 gr fresh/frozen snowpeas
- 1 bottle tomato sauce (freeze leftover)
- 1 small jar capers (optional)
- 4 (organic) tomatoes
- 1 pint grape/cherry tomatoes
- 2 lemons/limes
- 2 avocados
- 100 gr wild smoked salmon
- 1 cucumber
- 2 carrots
- 5 bell peppers
- 2 large containers of plain (Greek) yoghurt

- 1 jar of olives (optional)
- 1 small piece of feta
- 100 gr (3 oz) mushrooms
- 1 lb raw walnuts, pecans and almonds together
- 100 gr stir-fry beef
- 1 bunch of 2-3 broccoli heads/stems
- 1 bunch green onions
- 250 gram ground beef
- 1 bunch parsley
- 1 bunch cilantro (optional)
- 2 chicken thighs
- 6 apples (organic)
- 2 banana (organic)
- 1 bag frozen blueberries
- 3 oranges
- ½ cup almond flour
- 1/3 cup instant rolled oats
- 1/3 cup whole wheat flour
- ½ cup quinoa
- 100 gr extra dark chocolate (min 70% cacao)
- 1 liter buttermilk

Basic Spices and Herbs to Stock in your cupboard

- Salt
- Pepper
- Paprika
- rosemary, oregano, thyme, basil
- Organic soy sauce and/or coconut aminos (health food store, soy free
- alternative for soy sauce)
- nutmeg
- Thai fish sauce
- red pepper flakes

- onion powder
- garlic powder
- cayenne pepper
- sesame seed
- cinnamon
- maple syrup
- shredded coconut (unsweetened)
- coconut oil
- butter
- eggs
- garlic
- fresh ginger
- tomato paste
- tomato sauce
- frozen (blue) berries
- onions
- Plain or plain Greek yoghurt
- flaxseed (keep in fridge)
- brown rice
- baking powder
- baking soda
- small package of whole wheat flour (keep in fridge)
- instant rolled oats

Grocery Shopping List (Buy Non-Processed, Organically Grown)

Vegetables
Asparagus, Bean Sprouts, Beets, Bell Peppers, Bok Choy, Broccoli, Br. Sprouts, Cauliflower, Cabbage, Carrots, Celery, Cilantro, Cucumber, Eggplant, Garlic, Jalapeno Pep., Kale, Lettuce

Fruit
Low Glucose and Fructose
Limes, Lemon, Avocado, Cranberries, Pass. Fruit, Prune, Apricot, Cantaloupe, Raspberries, Plum, Kiwi, Blackberries, Cherries, Strawberries, Pineapple, Grapefruit

Grains
High Sugars
Amaranth, Barley, Brown Rice, Buckwheat, Oatmeal, Quinoa, Rye

Wheat Free
Almond Flour, Coconut Flour

Seeds
Chia, Hemp

Meat/Fowl
Bacon, Beef, Ground Beef, Stew Beef, Chicken, Chicken Breast, Chicken Wings, Chicken Liver, Duck, Ham, Kidney, Lamb, Pork, Sausage, Spare Rib, Steak, Turkey, Turk. Breast

Seafood
Anchovy, Catfish, Clam, Cod, Crab, Haddock, Halibut, Lobster, Mackerel, Mussel, oyster, Salmon (wild), Sardines, Scallop, Shrimp (wild), Snail, Squid, Trout

Dairy
Cheddar, Cottage Cheese, Cream, Sour Cream, Whipped Cream, Eggs, Feta, Milk, Mozzarella, Parmesan, Yogurt, Greek Yogurt

Legumes
Beans, Lentils, Peas

Oils
Almond Butter, Butter, Coconut Oil, Olives, Olive Oil, Peanut Butter

Raw Nuts
Almonds, Cashew, Chestnut, Macadamia, Peanut, Pecan, Pistachio, Pumpkin, Sesame, Sunflower

Leafy Greens
Mushrooms
Onions
Parsley
Pumpkin
Radish
Squash
Shallots
Spinach
Sweet Potato
Tomatoes
Turnip
White Potato
Yams
Zucchini

Tangerines
Pomegranate

Mod. Glucose and Fructose
Nectarines
Peach
Orange
Papaya
Banana
Blueberries
Dates
Apple

High Glucose and Fructose
Watermelon
Pears
Raisins
Grapes
Mango
Figs

Spices Etc.
Almond Milk
Apple Cider
Basil
Bay-leaves
Beef Bouillon
Chicken Bouillon
Capers
Cardamom
Cayenne
Chili Powder
Chili Sauce
Cinnamon
Cocoa
Coconut Milk
Coriander
Cumin
Curry Powder
Fennel Seeds
Garlic (powder)

Veal

Spices Etc.
Ginger
Mustard
Nutmeg
Onion Powder
Oregano
Paprika powder
Parsley
Pepper
Red Pep. Flakes
Rosemary
Sage
Salt
Thai Fish Sauce
Thyme
Turmeric
Tomato Sauce
Tomato Paste
Vanilla Extract
Vinegar

Tuna

Beverages
Coffee
Coffee Filters
Tea
Bottled Water

Alcohol
Beer
Red Wine
White Wine

Sweeteners
Xylitol
Maple Syrup
Honey

Walnuts

Household
Bathroom Cleaner
Count. Top Cloths
Detergent
Dish Washer Soap
Floor Cleaner
Floor Cloths
Foil Aluminium
Foil Plastic
Freezer Bags
Garbage Bags
Glass Cleaner
Laundry Detergent
Napkins
Oven Cleaner
Paper Towels
Sandwich Bags
Sponges/Scrubb.
Wax Paper
White Vinegar

Health/Beauty
Bath Soap
Body Lotion
Conditioner
Cosmetics
Cleaner/Tissues
Deodorant
Floss
Hair Gel
Hand Soap
Lip Balm
Mouthwash
Q-Tips
Razors
Shampoo
Shaving Cream
Shower Gel
Tampons
Toilet Paper
Toothpaste

"Brain & Body Fit After Forty"

Food and Fluid Journal

Meal	Monday	Tuesday	Wed.day	Thursday	Friday	Saturday	Sunday
Feeling: **Breakfast** Body Resp.							
Feeling: **Snack** Body Resp.							
Feeling: **Lunch** Body Resp.							
Feeling: **Snack** Body Resp.							
Feeling: **Dinner** Body Resp.							
Feeling: **Snack** Body Resp.							

"Brain & Body Fit After Forty"

Checklist for Achieving and Maintaining a Healthy Weight

- **Quality**
- **Quantity**
- **Timing**
- **Balance**
- **Mastering Your Eating Habits**

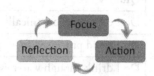

The five circles <u>together</u> and regular exercising form the foundation for physical and mental balance.

Establishing healthy eating and drinking habits is only possible by working on the five circles simultaneously. Leave one out and you are likely to go off track. Compare it to driving a car. If you don't pay attention to holding the steering wheel, other traffic, road- and weather conditions, signs, etcetera all at the same time, it is quite likely that you will never reach your destination.

Your body is not a machine and it won't always agree with what you want it to do. Weight loss is not an overnight thing and won't be a smooth journey either. You may plan to lose one or two pounds each week but your body follows its own schedule and may actually go faster, slower, come to a standstill or even go backwards for some time.

What If Things Don't Go As Planned.

Whatever happens, relax and focus on positive thoughts. Everybody hits a plateau at some point at which it seems impossible to get the body moving again. Simply sit down and figure out what is going on. Make it a challenge and have fun with it. Find out what works for you. The answer lies within you. Below you will find a checklist that covers all of the five circles.

See it as a tool to discover what more you can do to achieve your goals. Go from circle to circle, check your actions and see where you can make improvements.

Quality	√
Do I eat whole, organically grown non-processed food?	
Do I avoid processed food, fast food, convenience food?	
Do I drink enough water every day and don't drink soft drinks/sodas?	
Do I limit myself to 1 glass of alcohol per day?	
Quantity	**√**
Do I eat from a 9" plate; 1/3 protein, 2/3 non-starchy vegetables?	
Do I eat about 20 percent less than I usually do?	
Do I eat slowly and consciously and don't combine eating with other activities?	
Do I refrain from drinking when eating?	
Do I lay down my fork after every bite and take time to chew and taste?	
Do I leave the dishes in the kitchen?	
Do I listen to my body and know when enough is enough?	
Do I slow down breathing before eating and maintain slow breathing when eating?	
Do I keep a food and fluid journal?	
Do I practice daily the Step-One technique prolonged pointed attention?	
Timing	**√**
Do I eat 5 to 6 small meals every day?	
Do I start my days with a good breakfast?	
Do I plan my meals for the week ahead?	
Do I avoid shopping on an empty stomach?	
Do I avoid going to a party or other event on an empty stomach?	
Balance	**√**
Do I focus on eating vegetables and healthy fats when I'm not physically active?	
Do I eat complex carbohydrates about an hour prior to high impact activities?	
Do I avoid food and drinks my body can't digest well?	
Do I monitor my body responses after eating a meal or snack?	

Mastering Your Eating Habits	√
Do I practice daily the Step-Two technique vivid creative imagination and listen to the affirmations?	
Do I maintain an ongoing routine of Focus – Action – Reflection?	
Exercise	√
Do I regularly review the checklist optimizing results training program?	

"Brain & Body Fit After Forty"

Checklist Optimizing Results Training Program

- Fundamental Laws of Strength Training
- The Principles of Strength Training
- The six-Step Effective Exercise Plan
- The Full Body Workout
- Mastering Your Exercise Habits

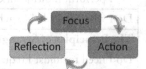

The 5 circles <u>together</u> and Healthy Nutrition form the foundation for physical balance.

Building a healthy and strong body is only possible by working on the five circles simultaneously. Leave one out and you are likely to go off track. Compare it to driving a car. If you don't pay attention to holding the steering wheel, other traffic, road- and weather conditions, signs, etcetera all at the same time, it is quite likely that you will never reach your destination.

Your body is not a machine and it won't always agree with what you want it to do. Building a strong physique is not an overnight thing and won't be a smooth journey either. You may plan to increase your strength every week but your body follows its own schedule and may actually go faster, slower or plateau at any time.

What If Things Don't Go As Planned.

Whatever happens, relax and focus on positive thoughts. Everybody hits a plateau at some point at which it seems impossible to get the body moving again. Simply sit down and figure out what is going on. Make it a challenge and have fun with it. Find out what works for you. The answer lies within you. Below you will find a checklist that covers all of the five circles. See it as a tool to discover what more you can do to achieve your goals. Go from circle to circle, check your actions and see where you can make improvements.

The Fundamental Laws of Strength Training	√
Do I work on enhancing joint flexibility?	
Do I work on Improving ligament and tendon strength?	
Do I work on Improving core strength?	
Do I work on Improving the strength of stabilizing muscles?	
Do I perform multi-joint exercises more than single joint exercises?	
Do I what is needed to achieve the set goals?	
The Principles of Strength Training	√
Do I need to adjust Frequency, Intensity, Time, Type?	
Am I ready to increase the resistance following the principle of progressive overload?	
Do I need to vary my workout program?	
Do I apply the principle of Individualization?	
Do I apply the principle of specificity?	
The Six-Step Effective Exercise Plan	√
Did I thoroughly answer the questions of the plan?	
Did I create a starting point?	
Did I design a sound program?	
Did I take action and workout consistently?	
Do I practice daily the Step-One technique prolonged pointed attention?	
The Full Body Workout	√
Do I follow workout guidelines?	
Do I keep track of my results in a workout journal?	
Do I vary my workouts?	
Do I work the entire metabolic system?	
Mastering Your Exercise Habits	√
Do I practice daily the Step-Two technique vivid creative imagination and listen to the affirmations?	
Do I maintain an ongoing routine of Focus – Action – Reflection?	
Healthy Nutrition	√
Do I regularly review the checklist achieving and maintaining a healthy weight?	

"Brain & Body Fit After Forty" Workout Journal Week...............

Exercises	Variations	Weight(s)	Sets	Reps	Comments
Legs	Squat Wide Stance	.......X.......	....	X	
	Squat Shoulder Width Stance	.......X.......	....	X	
	Squat Narrow Stance	.......X.......	....	X	
Chest	Regular Pushup	.......X.......	....	X	
	Modified Pushup	.......X.......	....	X	
	Chest Press	.......X.......	....	X	
Back	Row	.......X.......	....	X	
	Row-Clean and Press	.......X.......	....	X	
	Good Morning	.......X.......	....	X	
Biceps	Biceps Curl	.......X.......	....	X	
	Concentration Curl	.......X.......	....	X	
Triceps	Extension	.......X.......	....	X	
	Close Grip Bench Press	.......X.......	....	X	
	Dumbbell Kick Back		....	X	
Legs	Lunges	.......X.......	....	X	
Shoulders	Rear deltoids	2 X..........	....	X	
	Medial Deltoids	2 X..........	....	X	
	Front Deltoids	2 X.......	....	X	
	Shoulder Press	2 X.......	....	X	
Core	Abdominal Crunch		....	X	
	Crunch, Knees Bent		....	X	
	Leg raise		....	X	
	Oblique Crunch		....	X	
	Oblique Side Crunch		....	X	
	Plank		....	X	
	Side Plank		....	X	

"Brain & Body Fit After Forty"

Life Style Change Goal-Setting Plan and Journal

Your Healthy Nutrition and Effective Exercise Plan

---

1. **Is the goal specific, realistic and positive?**

2. **Why do I want what I want and what are the obstacles I can expect?**

3. **When will I know that I have achieved my goals?**

4. **What conditions are necessary to realize my goals?**

5. **Do I have what I need to achieve my goals?**

6. **Are the goals I want to achieve in alignment with my intentions in life?**

Your Healthy Nutrition and Effective Exercise Journal Describing the Successes and Challenges on Your Way Toward Your Goals.

Go by the five circles of both the Nutrition Part and the Exercise Part and follow for each of the circles the Focus – Action – Reflection routine.

Image: focus-action-reflection

Eating for Life	*Moving for Life*
Quality	Fundamental Laws of Strength Training
Quantity	Principles of Strength Training
Timing	The Six-Step Effective Exercise Plan
Balance	The Full Body Workout
Mastering Your Eating Habits	Mastering Your Exercise Habits

- Write in your journal at least once a week, following the format below.
- Begin with a positive experience, no matter how small or big.
- What aspect did you focus on and what were your actions and reflections?
- What are your successes and challenges?
- What are your strategies and actions for the coming days and week?

Todays' Date:

Positive Experience:

Past week's Focus, Actions and Reflections for:

Eating For Life / Moving For Life:

Successes and Challenges:

Strategies and Actions for the Coming Week:

Printed in the United States
By Hoof masters

Printed in the United States
By Bookmasters